Clinical Allergy and
Immunology of the Eye

**This volume is one of the series
Handbooks in Ophthalmology
Edited by Walter S. Schachat**

Other books in this series include:

Klein and Katzin: Microsurgery of the Vitreous
Meltzer: Ophthalmic Plastic Surgery for the General Ophthalmologist
Thompson: Topics in Neuro-ophthalmology
Charles: Vitreous Microsurgery
Carr and Siegel: Visual Electrodiagnostic Testing: A Practical Guide for
the Clinician

Clinical Allergy and Immunology of the Eye

Frederick H. Theodore, M.D.

Emeritus Clinical Professor of Ophthalmology,
Mount Sinai School of Medicine
Attending Ophthalmic Surgeon and
Director, External Disease and Infections Clinic,
Manhattan Eye, Ear and Throat Hospital
Consultant Ophthalmologist, The Mount Sinai Hospital
and Lenox Hill Hospital
New York, New York

Stephen E. Bloomfield, M.D.

Associate Professor of Ophthalmology, Cornell University Medical Center
Associate Scientist, Sloan-Kettering Institute
Assistant Attending Ophthalmologist, Manhattan Eye, Ear and Throat Hospital
Director, Cornea Clinic, The New York Hospital
New York, New York

Bartly J. Mondino, M.D.

Associate Professor of Ophthalmology,
Jules Stein Eye Institute, UCLA School of Medicine
Los Angeles, California

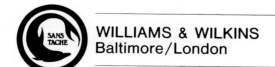

WILLIAMS & WILKINS
Baltimore/London

Copyright ©, 1983
Williams & Wilkins
428 East Preston Street
Baltimore, MD 21202, U.S.A.

Made in the United States of America

Library of Congress Cataloging in Publication Data

Theodore, Frederick H.
   Clinical allergy and immunology of the eye.

   (Handbooks in ophthalmology)
   Includes index.
   1. Eye—Diseases and defects—Immunological aspects. 2. Allergy. I. Bloomfield,
Stephen E. II. Mondino, Bartly, J. III. Title. IV. Series. [DNLM: 1. Eye—diseases—
Immunology. WW 160 T388c]
   RE69.T45 1983   617.7   82-13685
   ISBN 0-683-08175-6

Composed and printed at the
Waverly Press, Inc.
Mt. Royal and Guilford Aves.
Baltimore, MD 21202, U.S.A.

Preface

Physicians and other scientific investigators have long recognized the ever increasing importance of allergy and other immune mechanisms in the causation of eye diseases. In fact, by 1914—8 years after the term "Allergie" was first used by von Pirquet—von Szily had already published an ophthalmic text entitled *Die Anaphylaxie in der Augenheilkunde*. This is not surprising, because even at that time the eye and its adnexae offered a unique opportunity to observe and study, both clinically and experimentally, most fundamental immune reactions to an extent not possible elsewhere in the body until a much later date.

Clinical Allergy and Immunology of the Eye attempts to present a balanced clinical and practical view of the current understanding of the eye problems caused by abnormalities of the immune system based on the authors' long-term interests in ocular allergy, immunology, microbiology, and therapeutics. Until recently, immunology has been viewed by the practicing clinician as a rather esoteric and somewhat intimidating laboratory science. In a very short space of time the science, in all its ramifications, has leaped center stage, from laboratory into the clinical arena, with important practical applications for the physician in areas of diagnosis and treatment.

This monograph has three parts. The first three chapters deal with the elaboration of basic immune mechanisms, pathological immune reactions, and principles of treatment based on manipulating the immune response. These chapters have been diagrammatically illustrated in detail in order to give greater understanding to inherently difficult material.

The second part represents the major portion of the book and is essentially clinical, offering an application of the science of immunology to those clinical problems that the ophthalmologist must confront in his daily practice. In preparing this portion, it was gratifying to note how the basic allergic classifications and the ocular allergic phenomena described and delineated in our previous contributions are still valid today and form the framework of much of the book.

The third part is a glossary of terms, to again allow a quick reference for understanding the new and extensive terminology of immune science.

A number of illustrations used in this text were first printed in Theodore and Schlossman's *Ocular Allergy* published by Williams & Wilkins, Baltimore, 1958. The authors wish to thank both Dr. Abraham Schlossman and the publishers for permission to do so. They also wish to express their appreciation to Carlos Lopez, Ph.D., of the Sloan-Kettering Institute, for his editorial help in the preparation of the first portion of the manual. We also wish to express our appreciation to the American Academy of Ophthalmology for the use of material previously published in the Academy manual *Allergy of the Eye* by Dr. Theodore.

F.H.T.
S.E.B.
B.J.M.

Contents

SECTION ONE
BASIC CONCEPTS

Chapters 1–3

SECTION TWO
CLINICAL ASPECTS

Chapters 4–11

SECTION THREE
GLOSSARY

Chapter 12

CHAPTER ONE

Basic Immune Mechanisms

Protection from disease results from the detection and subsequent elimination of substances recognized as foreign by the immune system. This active protection against "non-self" is called immunity. Historically, the word derives from the Latin "immunitas," meaning freedom from taxes, and it later came to be used to indicate freedom from disease. The ancients realized that, after recovering from a disease, an individual was less susceptible to a recurrence of that disease. Modern immunology is the study of those systems responsible for protection of the individual against external and internal assault.

Foreign substances which have the capacity to evoke immunological responses are referred to as antigens. Antigens generally come from the external environment and include microbial organisms such as bacteria, viruses, and fungi. Plant, food, and animal products may also give rise to an immune response. Vaccines, drugs, and chemicals (such as food additives, dyes, and metals) may stimulate an immune reaction if introduced into a competent host. All antigens share the common characteristic of being recognized as foreign.

The immune system may also be activated by foreign substances from the internal environment, e.g., modified self-components such as virally infected cells or transformed (cancer) cells. However, if an immune response occurs against the host's own tissues, it is referred to as an autoimmune reaction.

Antigens range in size from the simplest low molecular weight molecules to the most complex microbial agents. Many antigens occurring in nature are substances of high molecular weight and usually are proteins or carbohydrates. By definition, immunogens are capable of inducing an immune response and of binding to the antibody directed against antigenic structural determinants found on the immunogen. Some small molecules cannot induce an immune response but bear antigenic determinants capable of binding antibody. These low molecular weight molecules, known as haptens, require prior attachment to a carrier protein in order to be immunogenic. Antigenic determinants are three-dimensional structures on the surface of immunogens which bind specific antibody. Most of the complex antigens, such as bacteria and red blood cells, contain numerous antigenic determinants.

Although immune responses generally result in elimination of foreign antigens without injury to the host, some antigens, referred to as allergens, may induce a hypersensitivity (allergic) reaction. The word allergy was coined in 1906 by von Pirquet to describe a state of altered reactivity. Today, the term is generally used to describe an acquired hypersensitivity which results in nonspecific damage to host tissue. In other words, allergy is a deleterious by-product of an immune response triggered by a foreign substance (allergen). Also implied is the fact that the allergen is usually innocuous, and its source is the external environment, e.g., pollens.

Occasionally, exposure to certain foreign antigenic determinants results in an unresponsive state referred to as immunological tolerance. Studies suggest that an active immune response mediated by suppressor T-cells may be responsible for this lack of reactivity. While a positive immune response results in elimination of the foreign substance, a negative response may be required to protect the host from allergic or autoantigenic responses. The balance between positive and negative reactivities determines whether or not an immune response is detectable. Tolerance may also be attained through the elimination of a responsive clone of lymphocytes, i.e., clonal deletion.

IMMUNE RESPONSE

The immune response (Fig. 1.1) is a complex sequence of events in which the host recognizes that foreign molecules are invading the system (afferent arc) and then mobilizes a reaction against them (efferent arc). There are two types of responses which can occur, a nonspecific response and a specific response. The progression of these responses depends on the nature of the antigen and the genetic constitution of the host.

Nonspecific Response

The reticuloendothelial system (RES), a phylogenetically primitive system, mediates the host's nonspecific response. This system requires no prior experience with the foreign material and, therefore, expresses no immunological memory. The cells of the RES, macrophages, monocytes, and granulocytes effect inflammatory responses and the phagocytosis and clearing of foreign particles. Since this is a first encounter, there is no pre-existing antibody to facilitate engulfment of foreign particles. The RES effects removal of particulate substances such as certain bacteria and parasites.

The natural killer (NK) cell system (Fig. 1.2) is a newly described effector of resistance against virus-infected and tumor cells. The cells which mediate this response are marrow-dependent and, although not macrophages, appear to be re-

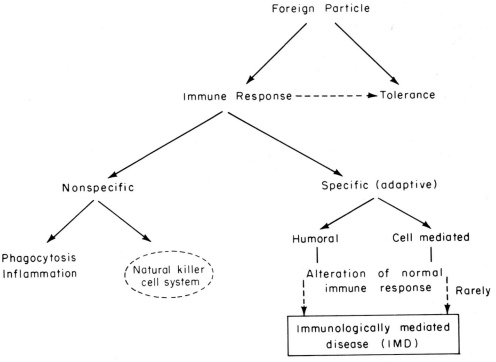

Figure 1.1 Possible reaction to foreign particle. Encounter with a foreign antigen (for example, a virus) could result in unresponsiveness to that antigen (tolerance) but, most likely, it would lead to both a non-specific and a specific (adaptive) immune response. Although the combination of humoral and cell-mediated immune responses would probably clear the antigen, it might persist and its stimulation of the immune response might result in immunologically mediated disease.

lated to the macrophage/neutrophil lineage of cells.

Specific Adaptive Immune Response

During the primary encounter with antigen, macrophages process and present antigen to other cells of the immune system. The latter then mediate the specific or adaptive immune response (Fig. 1.3). This system is phylogenetically more recently developed than nonspecific immunity and also differs in expressing specificity and memory. The two major responses elicited in the adaptive immune response are humoral and cell-mediated immunity. These two responses are primarily mediated by different subpopulations of lymphocytes. The cell-mediated immune response is mediated by thymus-derived cells (T-cells). The humoral immune response is mediated by B-cells (bursa-derived in chickens, or its bone marrow equivalent in humans), but it also requires some T-cell participation.

Recent studies suggest that the macrophage plays a central role in various aspects of the adaptive immune response.[1-3] Macrophages process antigen and present it (in conjunction with cellular determinants) to the appropriate lymphocyte populations and are also capable of modulating these responses by the production and secretion of helper and suppressor factors.

Nonspecific and adaptive immunity are complemented and enhanced by the Biological Amplification System: the coagulation-kinin sequence and the complement cascade. All of these could be included as part of the nonspecific response, while activation of complement by the classical pathway (by antigen-antibody complexes) could be included as part of the adaptive immune response.

HUMORAL IMMUNITY

Three cell populations, macrophages, T-cells, and B-cells, must interact in order for antigen stimulation to result in an antibody response to most naturally occurring antigens (Fig. 1.4). The antigen is processed by the macrophages and then presented as part of its cell surface in association with self-determinants to the lymphoid cells. The presentation of antigen to the B-cells in conjunction with T-cell help (probably by way of a helper factor induced by interaction of helper T-cell with antigen) results in the transformation of B-cells into a large, metaboli-

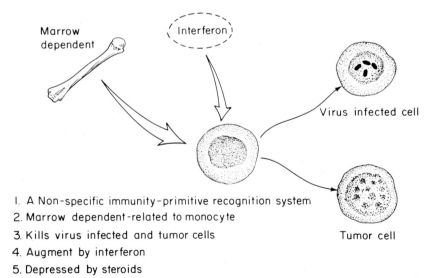

Marrow dependent

Interferon

Virus infected cell

Tumor cell

1. A Non-specific immunity-primitive recognition system
2. Marrow dependent-related to monocyte
3. Kills virus infected and tumor cells
4. Augment by interferon
5. Depressed by steroids

Figure 1.2   Natural killer (NK) cell system. The NK cell system is thought to play an important role in resistance to syngeneic tumors and virus infections. The effector cell is dependent on the bone marrow for maturation and appears to be related to the macrophage/neutrophil lineage. Interferon augments NK cell function and may be required for NK cell activity.

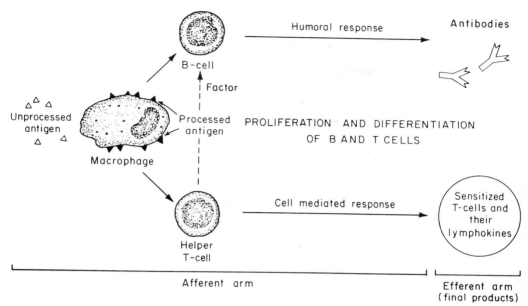

Figure 1.3 Basic organization of adaptive immunity. Macrophages, B-cells, and T-cells interact in the generation of an adaptive immune response. Antigen is processed by the macrophage and presented to the T-cells and B-cells, with the help of a factor made by T-cells, producing antibodies, the effector molecules of the humoral immune response. T-cell subpopulations interact to produce sensitized lymphocytes which effect cell-mediated immunity.

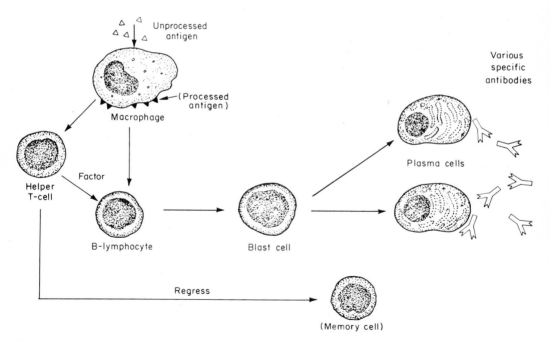

Figure 1.4 Humoral immune response. The humoral immune response requires the presentation of processed antigen by the macrophage to the B-cells. Macrophages present antigen in the context of self antigen to T-cells which then produce a factor which helps B-cells differentiate to produce antibody.

cally active "blast cells," which then differentiate into plasma cells that produce antibody. Burnet's clonal selection theory proposes that antigen reacts with pre-existing receptors on B-lymphocytes, leading to proliferation and activation of those cells.

On first stimulation with antigen, the host produces IgM antibodies while a second exposure to antigen or continued exposure, as in a virus infection, results in an IgG antibody response. The response to a second exposure to antigen, referred to as an anamnestic response, is faster and stronger than the first response. This is a function of memory T-cells. They are a subpopulation of sensitized T-cells which regress to small lymphocytes. These memory cells then proliferate and promote both the strong secondary response and the conversion to IgG production.

The mechanisms which result in the great diversity of specificities of antibody capable of binding with the very large number of different antigenic determi-nants are being defined at the molecular level. Briefly, this great diversity is generated by the rearrangement of a number of genes which code for the various portions of the immunoglobulin molecules. The choice of the genetic regions (from among many), as well as the way in which they are spliced together, results in the many possible antigen binding sites.

The humoral immune response to certain linear antigens such as pneumococcal polysaccharide and endotoxin is T-cell independent. This response also appears to be independent of macrophage processing and presentation and probably depends on a stimulatory effect of this type of antigen on B-cells.

Antibody: Structure and Function

Antibodies are found in the globulin fraction of the serum and are referred to as immunoglobulins (Ig). The basic Ig molecule is made up of two light polypeptide chains (L) and two heavy chains (H) held together by disulfide bridges (Fig. 1.5).

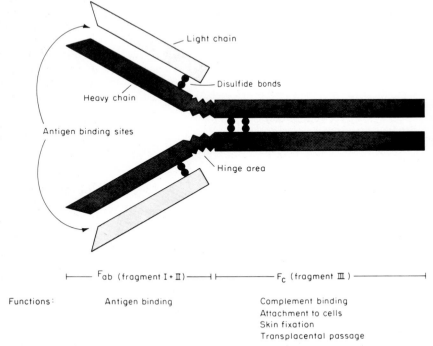

Figure 1.5 Schematic representation of basic antibody molecule consisting of two light chains and two heavy chains held together by disulfide bonds. The two Fab fragments contain the antigen binding sites. The Fc fragment is responsible for binding complement, attaching to cells, fixing to skin, and transplacental passage.

The L-chains for all Ig molecules are of two kinds—lambda and kappa—while the H-chains of each immunoglobulin class are different and determine the Ig class. The basic Ig molecule assumes a Y shape: the upper arms are each composed of an L-chain and part of an H-chain, and the tail is made up of the rest of the two H-chains. The fragments which contain the antibody binding sites (Fab) are in the small arms; each Ig molecule contains two Fabs. The tail, referred to as the Fc portion because it is the crystallizable fragment, is responsible for many of the other properties of the Ig molecules, such as complement activation and binding to phagocytes.

Analysis of the structure of the Fab portion of the Ig molecule indicates that both the L-chain and the H-chain have amino acid sequences which are the same from one molecule to the next (constant regions), while certain sequences are variable. When the Ig molecule folds into its normal three-dimensional configuration, hypervariable segments form the antigen binding site. The variability of amino acid sequences results in variable three-dimensional binding sites which conform to the antigen and thus result in the specificity of the antibody for antigen.

Immunoglobulin G (IgG)

IgG is the most abundant Ig in the serum and the predominant Ig in the eye. It has a molecular weight (M.W.) of 150,000 and is the only Ig to cross the placenta. There are four subclasses of IgG determined by different H-chains. The different H-chains bestow slightly different biological properties to each subclass, e.g., the capacity to bind complement or the ability to block IgE binding.

During a nonspecific response, macrophages and neutrophils phagocytose foreign particles such as bacteria which adhere weakly to nonspecific sites on the surface of the phagocytes. This activity is greatly enhanced during the adaptive immune response due to the cytophilic nature of IgG. The exposed Fab sites of IgG antibodies or opsonins combine with the antigen (bacteria), and the Fc portions of the antibodies adhere to Fc receptors on the surface of phagocytic cells, thereby enhancing phagocytosis. Both opsonization and a second phenomenon, immune adherence, facilitate clearing of antigen by phagocytic cells (Fig. 1.6). Immune adherence results from the activation of complement by the interaction of antigen with IgG or IgM. One complement component bound to the antigen-antibody complexes, C3b, increases binding to phagocytes through their C3b receptors; this results in increased phagocytosis.

Immunoglobulin A (IgA)

IgA is the dominant Ig found in external secretions and is thus referred to as the secretory Ig. It is also found in the serum, where it is the second most abundant Ig. In serum, IgA is present as a monomer of M.W. 160,000, similar to IgG, but in secretions it is found as a dimer linked by a small polypeptide chain and a secretory component (SC). The SC is produced by epithelial cells and is attached to IgA as it is transported across the mucous membrane (Fig. 1.7). The SC appears to protect the IgA molecule from enzymatic degradation and also helps fix it to the mucosa. The lacrimal gland has IgA-producing plasma cells in it, SC-producing epithelial cells in its acini, ducts and tubules, and secretory IgA in the tears bathing its mucosal surface.[4] SC has also been found in conjunctival epithelium.[5] IgA plays an important role in defense against infection of mucous membranes, coating microorganisms to prevent their adherence to mucosal cells. IgA also has the ability to activate complement by the alternative pathway.

Immunoglobulin M (IgM)

IgM (M.W. 900,000) is the largest of the immunoglobulins and is made up of five monomers held together by a small polypeptide and disulfide bridges (Fig. 1.8). On primary exposure to an antigen, IgM antibodies are the first to be made. Biologically, IgM antibodies fix complement and agglutinate particulate antigen with a higher degree of efficiency than do other Ig's.

Immunoglobulin D (IgD)

IgD (M.W. 185,000) is found in very low concentrations in the serum. Because it

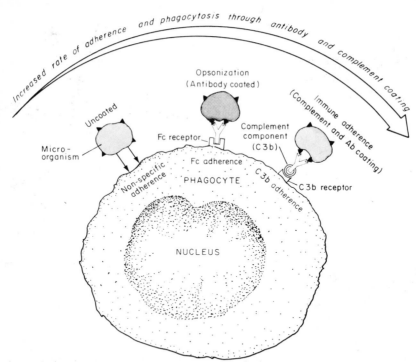

Figure 1.6 Antibody (opsonin) and complement facilitate phagocytosis of particles by enhancing their adherence to phagocytic cells. Immunoglobulin G attaches via an Fc receptor or complement C3b, fixed to an antibody molecule, attaches via the C3 receptor. Opsonization and immune adherence increase phagocytosis.

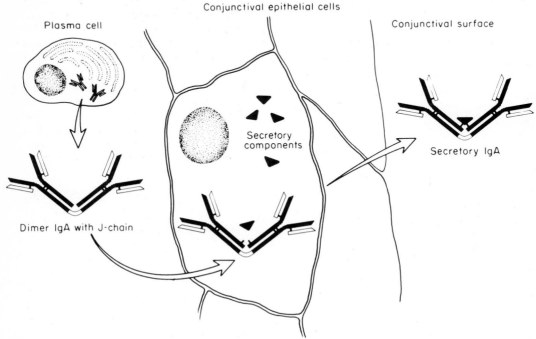

Figure 1.7 The secretory component (SC) is added to the IgA molecule as it is transported across mucous membranes, including the lacrimal gland and conjunctival epithelium.

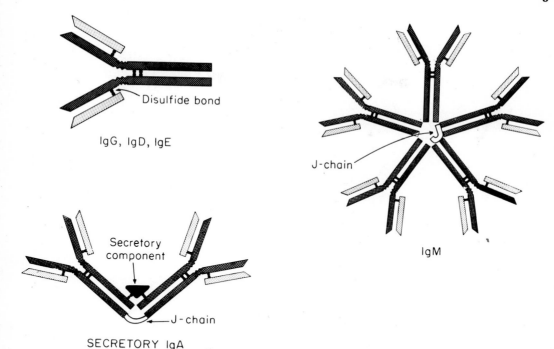

Figure 1.8 IgG, IgD, IgE, and serum IgA are all similar in structure: They are made up of the basic four-chain structure described for IgG. IgA in secretions is a dimer held together by a small J-piece. IgM is a pentamer held together by a J-piece and disulfide bonds.

has been found bound to the membrane of lymphocytes, it is thought that it may serve as a receptor for antigens.

Immunoglobulin E (IgE)

IgE (M.W. 200,000) is present in serum in minute concentrations. Levels of IgE are markedly elevated in patients with atopic allergy. The combination of IgE and allergen, while the IgE is bound to mast cells or basophils, causes degranulation and release of vasoamines which are responsible for allergic reactions (Fig. 1.9). IgE may also play a role in defense against certain parasitic infections.

Immunoglobulins have been found in all structures of the eye except the lens.[6] The highest concentrations were found in the cornea, choroid, and conjunctiva. All five immunoglobulins and albumin were present in the immunoglobulin-containing tissues except for the cornea, which did not routinely contain IgM centrally. Although the concentration of IgG and IgA appears to be uniform throughout the cornea, significantly less IgM is found in the central than in the peripheral cornea,

probably because the large size of IgM restricts its diffusion into the cornea from the limbus.[7] Immunoglobulins in the human cornea are probably derived from the limbal vessels. The ocular surface epithelium is usually free of immunoglobulins and albumin.

The immunoglobulin with the highest concentration in tears is IgA followed by IgG.[8] The relative concentration of IgG increases in the tears with inflammation of the external eye probably from transudation of serum proteins from vessels of the external eye.

CELL-MEDIATED IMMUNE RESPONSE

As the name implies, the cell-mediated immune (CMI) response is mediated by cells, not by humoral factors. In experimental animals the capacity to produce a CMI response can be transferred by lymphoid cells, but not by serum. CMI responses are T-cell functions which do not require B-cells or antibody to be expressed (Fig. 1.10).

The CMI response mediates delayed-type hypersensitivity (DTH) reactions,

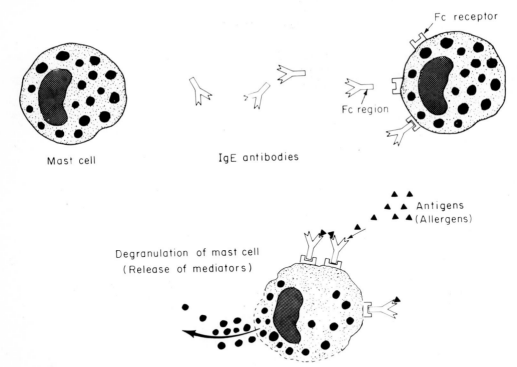

Figure 1.9 Schematic representation of mast cell degranulation. The Fc portion of the IgE molecule binds tightly to Fc receptor in cell surface. Binding by IgE of allergen results in degranulation of cell, release of various mediators, and symptoms of allergy.

skin (or other organ) graft rejection, and graft-versus-host (GvH) reactions in humans. An example of DTH reaction is the tuberculin test: prior exposure to *Mycobacterium tuberculosis* results in sensitized lymphocytes which migrate to the site of injected antigen, causing other cells to be attracted to the site. The accumulated cells present as a visible, palpable lump 48 hours after subcutaneous injection of antigen. Similarly, skin (or other organ) transplantation from a histoincompatible (non-twin) donor results in the sensitization of lymphoid cells, their migration to the site of the graft, and the killing of the grafted tissue by host lymphoid cells. GvH reactions, on the other hand, are the result of transplanting normal bone marrow cells into a histoincompatible host. Such a transfer leads to sensitization of the donated cells to host cells and the initiation of destructive reactivity against the host. In each of these reactions, a T-cell is the effector of the CMI response.

The mixed leukocyte culture (MLC) and the cell-mediated lympholysis (CML) reactions are two in vitro assays of CMI. As with the in vivo phenomena described above, the MLC and the CML are both mediated by T-cells. In fact, these in vitro models are thought to be good correlates of the in vivo phenomena. In the MLC assay, lymphocytes from one individual are cultured with lymphocytes from another individual who has been treated with x-rays or mitomycin C so that the lymphocytes are unable to proliferate. The T-cells become sensitized and proliferate in response to foreign determinants on the other population of lymphocytes. These lymphocyte activating determinants (Lad) are present mostly on B-cells, while the responding cells are predominantly T-cells. The proliferation is detected by the degree of incorporation of radioactive precursors into the sensitized cells. For the CML assay, similarly sensitized cells are evaluated for their capacity to kill cells of the type used to stimulate.

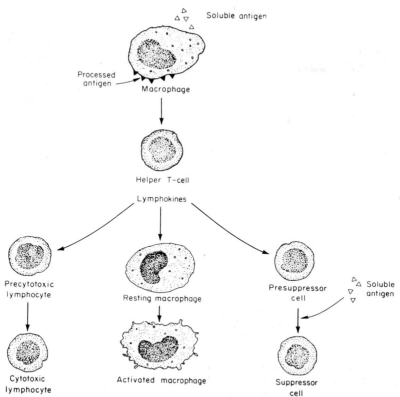

Figure 1.10 In the cell-mediated immune response, processed antigen is presented to T-cells in the context of self antigen. Helper T-cells proliferate and produce lymphokines which affect the functions of at least three subpopulations of cells: 1) precytotoxic T-cells become cytotoxic, 2) resting macrophages become activated, and 3) presuppressor cells become suppressor cells. Soluble antigen can also induce suppressor cells.

Cytotoxic lymphocytes kill histoincompatible target cells that are labeled with radioactive chromium, and killing is detected by the amount of chromium released into the fluid medium.

Several subpopulations of T-cells as well as macrophages are required for the CMI response[9] (Fig. 1.10). Macrophages process antigen and present it as a complex of processed antigen *plus* cell surface antigens. Although B-cells recognize antigen alone on the macrophage cell surface, T-cells recognize antigen only in conjunction with self-antigens. This is an important difference which can lead to different kinds of responses for certain antigens. Helper T-cells respond by proliferating and producing lymphokines which are soluble mediators of the CMI response. These lymphokines then affect three different cell populations. 1) Precy-totoxic lymphocytes are induced to become cytotoxic lymphocytes capable of killing cells which express the combination of foreign antigen and self-antigen presented by the macrophage (e.g., cytotoxic lymphocytes will kill "foreign" transplanted tissues or hosts cells made foreign by virus infection). 2) Certain lymphokines affect the function of macrophages (e.g., macrophages may be recruited to the site of infection and their capacity to phagocytose and kill microorganisms enhanced). 3) Lymphokines also act to induce suppressor T-cells. Suppressor cells can be antigen specific or nonspecific and can, in addition, be induced by soluble antigen. Suppressor cells have been shown to inhibit both cell-mediated and humoral immune responses and appear to play an important homeostatic role. Because a normal immune response can lead to inappropriate damage to normal cells, suppressor T-cells are considered vital in maintaining a balanced immune response and reducing this damage.

Role of the Macrophage

Macrophages are large phagocytic cells found fixed in tissues. Their precursors, monocytes, are present in the circulation (Fig. 1.11). These cells play a central role in the immune response.[1-3] They are absolutely required for the initiation of either a humoral or cell-mediated immune response since they process and present antigen to lymphoid cells in an immunogenic form (Fig. 1.12). Macrophages are also essential to the efferent limb of the immune response: antibody augments the capacity of these cells to phagocytose and clear bacterial pathogens, while lymphokines, produced as a result of the CMI response, augment the capacity of these cells to destroy tumor cells. A T-cell product "arms" the macrophages for killing target cells. Macrophages are "activated" when re-exposed to antigen and are then capable of nonspecifically killing target cells (Fig. 1.11). Macrophages have also been shown to elaborate factors which augment or suppress lymphocyte function and, may also serve a regulatory function.

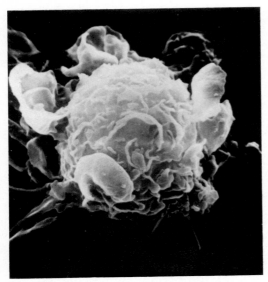

Figure 1.11 Scanning electronphotomicrograph of an activated macrophage. (Courtesy of John Hadden, M.D.)

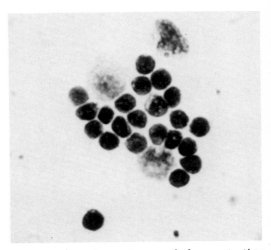

Figure 1.12 Photomicrograph demonstrating close relationship between larger macrophages and smaller lymphocytes. Macrophages process antigen and present it to the appropriate lymphocyte populations.

GENETICS OF THE IMMUNE RESPONSE

Since the basic function of the immune system is to recognize and eliminate foreign substances, the host must have a system for determining what is "self" and what is "non-self." Skin graft rejection and tumor immunity correlated with a cell surface antigen in certain inbred strains of mice has been demonstrated. A number of investigators have subsequently shown that this antigen, termed antigen II, was, in fact, the major histocompatibility system of the mouse. Antigen II is not actually a single antigen: it is a complex of many antigens encoded by a small region on the 17th chromosome of the mouse. This highly polymorphic, multigene complex has been renamed the H-2 (H-histocompatibility; 2-second antigen) complex and has been found to control a wide variety of immunological phenomena. An understanding of the H-2 complex and its function is central to understanding modern immunobiology.

All mammals have a major histocompatibility complex comparable to the mouse. In man, this complex is called the HLA system (Fig. 1.13), because of its initial discovery on human leukocytes (human leukocyte antigens—HLA). As found earlier in the mouse, the HLA complex

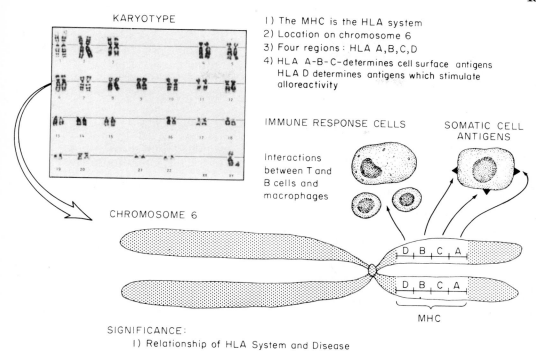

KARYOTYPE

1) The MHC is the HLA system
2) Location on chromosome 6
3) Four regions: HLA A,B,C,D
4) HLA A-B-C-determines cell surface antigens
   HLA D determines antigens which stimulate alloreactivity

IMMUNE RESPONSE CELLS   SOMATIC CELL ANTIGENS

Interactions between T and B cells and macrophages

CHROMOSOME 6

D B C A

D B C A

MHC

SIGNIFICANCE:
1) Relationship of HLA System and Disease
2) Modulation of Immune Response

Figure 1.13 Diagram illustrating the location and function of the major histocompatibility complex (MHC), the HLA, in humans.

can be divided into subregions, coding for antigens involved in different aspects of the immune response.[10] Three of the four major subregions, HLA-A, B and C, code for serologically defined cell surface antigens found on almost all body cells. These antigens, when they appear on any type of grafted tissue, can be recognized as non-self by the immune system of the host, resulting in graft rejection.

The HLA-D region of this complex codes for cell surface glycoproteins found on a limited repertoire of cells including B-cells, some macrophages, and a small subpopulation of T-cells. The products of the genetic region are thought to be involved in the presentation of foreign antigens by the macrophage to lymphoid cells. This presentation determines whether or not an immune response will be generated to simple antigens and the nature of that response. The gene products of the HLA-D region govern many of the important cellular interactions which regulate the immune response and have thus become a focus for study.

Each region of the HLA complex (A, B, C, and D) is a highly polymorphic, multiallelic family of genes. The specificities determined by these genes are described using naturally occurring antibodies found in the serum of multiparous women. The sum of the serologically determined specificities encoded in an individual makes up the HLA complex of that person.

Although historically the major histocompatibility complex was identified as a tissue recognition system to detect the potential of graft rejection, it is unlikely that this is its main biological function. Recent studies suggest that a major role for HLA may be in susceptibility or resistance to disease. Thus, in order for a virally infected host cell to be killed by cytotoxic lymphocytes, both viral and cellular (HLA-A, B, or C) antigens must be recognized. A more direct relationship between HLA and disease susceptibility has also been described: People with certain serologically determined HLA antigens have been found to have very high risks of developing certain diseases. For example, the HLA-B27 antigen has been found on cells from about 90% of patients with ankylosing spondylitis. Currently these studies are helpful in the diagnosis of certain diseases; eventually they may help in the understanding of the pathogenesis of these diseases.

BIOLOGICAL AMPLIFICATION SYSTEM

The coagulation-kinin cascade and the complement pathways serve to support and amplify both cell-mediated and humoral immune responses.

Coagulation-Kinin Cascade

The proteins of the coagulation-kinin cascade include Hageman factor (coagulation factor XII), prekallikrein, coagulation factor XI, plasminogen, and high molecular weight-kininogen (precursor of bradykinin).[11] They are proteolytic enzymes which are found in the blood as inactive precursors. Activation of these components occurs by partial proteolysis. The active products of these reactions can initiate biological effects such as coagulation, vasodilation, increased vascular permeability, fibrinolysis, and chemotaxis. Attracting phagocytic cells to an inflammatory focus appears to be critical for the immunologically mediated host defense against bacterial pathogens. Tissue injury secondary to some other mechanisms such as inflammation caused by deposition of immune complexes often precedes the participation of the coagulation-kinin cascade, which is often a later event in the inflammatory process.

Complement Cascade

Complement is a system of serum proteins that act in a specified sequence so that one component, when activated, activates several molecules of the next component so that a cascade effect with amplification is produced (Fig. 1.14). The classical pathway of complement depends upon the operation of nine protein components (C1–C9), with C1 being a trimolecular complex of three proteins termed C1q, C1r, and C1s. The classical pathway of complement activation depends on an antibody-antigen reaction. C1q, the recognition unit of the classical pathway, binds to the Fc portion of IgG or IgM bound to antigen. Activation of C1q leads to activation of classical pathway components in the following sequence: C1r, C1s, C4, C2, and C3. The most critical step in the complement system is the proteolytic cleavage of C3 to C3a and C3b by complement enzymes termed "C3 convertases."[12] Cleavage of C4 and C2 by $\overline{C1}$ (horizontal bar above complement component indicates activation) results in the production of the classical pathway C3 convertase, $\overline{C4b2a}$.

The alternative pathway of complement does not depend on an antibody-antigen reaction but is activated by aggregated IgA and microbial products such as endotoxin and zymosan. It can also be activated by a feedback loop mechanism from the classical pathway through C3b. The components of the alternative pathway include C3, factor B, factor D, and properdin. Participation of the early complement components (C1, C4, and C2) is not necessary for the alternative pathway. The stable C3 convertase of the alternative pathway, $\overline{C3bBb}$ (P), consists of C3b, factor B, and properdin (which serves to stabilize the enzyme).

The alternative pathway may be the very earliest host response to microbial infections and provides the nonimmune host with a type of antimicrobial defense that can operate during the time required for a specific immune response to develop.

After activation of C3, the pivotal complement component, the alternative and classical pathways are identical with activation of C5, C6, C7, C8, and C9.

Activated complement is the prime mediator of tissue inflammation. Functions of activated complement include the following:

1. Chemotaxis. The biologically active fragment C5a causes chemotaxis of polymorphonuclear leukocytes.

2. Anaphylatoxin activity. Biologically active fragments C3a and C5a cause histamine release from mast cells and basophils thereby resulting in vasodilation and increased vascular permeability. This provides an increased supply of plasma proteins including complement at the site of inflammation.

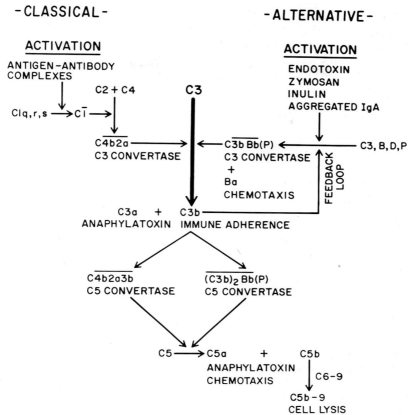

- CLASSICAL -

ACTIVATION

ANTIGEN-ANTIBODY
COMPLEXES

C2 + C4   C3

Clq,r,s ⟶ C$\overline{1}$ ⟶

C4b2a ⟶
C3 CONVERTASE

C3a + C3b
ANAPHYLATOXIN IMMUNE ADHERENCE

C4b2a3b
C5 CONVERTASE

- ALTERNATIVE -

ACTIVATION

ENDOTOXIN
ZYMOSAN
INULIN
AGGREGATED IgA

← C$\overline{3b}$ Bb(P) ←   ← C3, B, D, P
C3 CONVERTASE
+
Ba
CHEMOTAXIS

FEEDBACK LOOP

(C3b)$_2$ Bb(P)
C5 CONVERTASE

C5 ⟶ C5a + C5b
ANAPHYLATOXIN
CHEMOTAXIS   C6-9

C5b-9
CELL LYSIS

Figure 1.14 The complement cascade can be activated by antigen/antibody complexes (classical pathway) or by endotoxin, or aggregated IgA (the alternate pathway). Activation of complement releases biologically active mediators of chemotaxis and inflammation. Activation of the terminal components results in cell lysis.

3. Immune adherence. C3b is responsible for immune adherence. C3b in complexes with antigen and antibody binds to polymorphonuclear leukocytes and macrophages which have specific receptors on their membranes for C3b. This immune adherence facilitates subsequent phagocytosis.

4. Cytolysis. Activation of the full complement system through C9 by either the classical or alternative pathway may lead to membrane damage and cell lysis. The membrane attack complex that punches holes in cell membranes consists of C5b, C6, C7, C8, and C9.

Normal human donor corneas have been shown to contain C1q, C3, C4, C5, properdin, and factor B using gel double diffusion.[13] In another study, functional C1, C4, C2, C3, C5, C6, and C7 were demonstrated and quantitated in normal human donor corneas using a hemolytic assay that depends on the ability of complement to cause lysis of red blood cells sensitized with antibodies.[14] For all seven of these complement components, hemolytic activities in the peripheral cornea were higher than hemolytic activities in the central cornea, suggesting that the major source of complement components is the limbal vessels and that complement components diffuse from the limbus to the central cornea.[15] The difference between hemolytic activities in the central and peripheral cornea was most striking for C1 (the recognition unit of the classical pathway and largest complement component). The large size of C1 may restrict its diffusion into the cornea, and this finding may be important in peripheral inflammation and ulcers of the cornea. Because of the function of C1 as the recognition unit of the classical pathway, antigen-antibody complexes, whether formed in the cornea itself or whether derived from the tears, aqueous humor, or limbal vessels, may activate complement more effectively in the peripheral than in the central cornea. Corneal fibroblasts have the ability to produce C1 in tissue culture but it is not known whether they are producing this complement component in vivo.[16]

Activation of complement by either the classical or alternative pathway may be involved in corneal inflammation.[17, 18] Using direct immunofluorescent techniques, components of both the classical and alternative pathway have been identified in rabbit and human corneas in association with microbial infections.

Hemolytic complement of both the classical and alternative pathways was found to be present in normal tears, suggesting that the complement pathways could be included among the defense mechanisms of the ocular surface.[19]

C4 has been detected in normal aqueous humor.[20] In addition to C4, C3 and C1 have been found in aqueous humor in patients with anterior segment inflammation.

IMMUNOLOGICALLY MEDIATED DISEASE

Although the immune response is required for protecting the host from the numerous pathogens found in the environment, this same immune system can cause damage to normal tissue (Fig. 1.1). Whether or not tissue damage occurs depends on the type of antigen, its location, and the nature of the immunological response of the host. Moreover, antigen must persist at the site of injury for the development of immunologically mediated disease. Four different types of reactions, triggered by humoral or cell-mediated immune response, may cause damage to normal tissues. Each of these types of reactions has a different mechanism of action and these mechanisms often interact when causing tissue injury. This is discussed in Chapter 2.

SUMMARY

The immune response protects the host from disease caused by pathogens from an external source. An invading pathogen first encounters the nonspecific resistance mechanism made up of phagocytic cells and NK cells. These systems are very primitive, require no previous experience with the invading microorganisms, and demonstrate no memory. Foreign antigens are concomitantly processed for development of the adaptive immune response. Adaptive immunity is phylogenetically less primitive, requires a previous encounter with an antigen to be expressed, and demonstrates memory. The two main arms of adaptive immunity are the humoral immune response, mediated by antibodies produced by B-lymphocytes, and the cell-mediated immune response, mediated by T-lymphocytes. Macrophages play a central role in these responses, since they are required for antigen processing and presentation, as well as being effector cells in the cell-mediated immune response. Many aspects of the adaptive immune response are governed by genes within the major histocompatibility complex, the HLA complex in humans. Genes within this relatively small region govern cellular interaction as well as host capacity to respond to certain antigens. The immune response is assisted and augmented by the biological amplification systems. These play a role in inflammation and chemotaxis. In addition, complement is an effector of humoral immunity. Although the immune response is required for protection of the host, these responses can also be harmful, causing damage to normal tissues.

REFERENCES

1. Rosenthal, A.S. Regulation of the immune response—Role of the macrophage. N. Engl. J. Med. 303:1153–1156, 1980.
2. Nathan, C.F., Murray, H.W., Cohn, Z.A. The macrophage as an effector cell. N. Engl. J. Med. 303:622–626, 1980.
3. Unanue, E.R. Cooperation between mononuclear phagocytes and lymphocytes in immunity. N. Engl. J. Med. 303:977–985, 1980.
4. Cohen, E.J., Allansmith, M.R. Fixation tech-

niques for secretory components in human lacrimal gland and conjunctiva. Am. J. Ophthalmol. 91:789–793, 1981.

5. Franklin, R.M., Prendergast, R.A., Silverstein, A.M. Secretory immune system of rabbit ocular adnexa. Invest. Ophthalmol. Visual Sci. 18:1093, 1979.

6. Allansmith, M.R., Whitney, C.R., McClellan, B.H., Newman, L.P. Immunoglobulins in the human eye. Arch. Ophthalmol 89:36–45, 1973.

7. Allansmith, M.R., McClellan, B.H. Immunoglobulins in the human cornea. Am. J. Ophthalmol. 80:123–132, 1975.

8. McClellan, B.S., Whitney, C.R., Newman, L.P., Allansmith, M.R. Immunoglobulins in tears. Am. J. Ophthalmol. 76:89–101, 1973.

9. Reinherz, E.L., Schlossman, S.F. Regulation of the immune response—Inducer and suppressor T-lymphocyte subsets in human beings. N. Engl. J. Med. 303: 370–373, 1980.

10. Mc Devitt, H.O. Regulation of the immune response by the major histocompatibility system. N. Engl. J. Med. 303:1514–1517, 1980.

11. Kaplan, A.P. The complement, coagulation and kinin-forming cascades in inflammation. Proceedings of Immunology of the eye. Workshop III, edited by Suran, A., Gery, I., and Nussenblatt, R.B. Immunology Abstr. (Suppl.) pp. 383–399, 1981.

12. Fearon, D.T., Austen, K.F. The alternative pathway of complement—A system for host resistance to microbial infection. N. Engl. J. Med. 303:259–263, 1980.

13. Mondino, B.J., Ratajczak, H.V., Goldberg, D.B., Schanzlin, D., Brown, S.I. Alternate and classical pathway components of complement in the normal cornea. Arch. Ophthalmol. 98:346–349, 1980.

14. Mondino, B.J., Hoffman, D.B. Hemolytic complement activity in normal human donor corneas. Arch. Ophthalmol. 98:2041–2044, 1980.

15. Mondino, B.J., Brady, K.J. Distributioin of hemolytic complement in the normal cornea. Arch. Ophthalmol. 99:1430–1433, 1981.

16. Mondino, B.J., Sundar-Raj, C.V., Brady, K.J. Production of C1 by corneal fibroblasts. Arch. Ophthalmol. 100:478–480, 1982.

17. Mondino, B.J., Rabin, B.S., Kessler, E., Gallo, J., Brown, S.I. Corneal rings with gram-negative bacteria. Arch. Ophthalmol. 92:2222–2225, 1977.

18. Mondino, B.J., Brown, S.I., Rabin, B.S., Bruno, J. Alternate pathway activation of complement in a *Proteus mirabilis* ulceration of the cornea. Arch. Ophthalmol. 96:1659–1661, 1978.

19. Yamamoto, G.K., Allansmith, M.R. Complement in tears from normal humans. Am. J. Ophthalmol. 88:758–763, 1979.

20. Chandler, J.W., Leder, R., Kaufman, H.E., Caldwell, J.R. Quantitative determinations of complement components and immunoglobulins in tears and aqueous humor. Invest. Ophthalmol. 13: 151–153, 1974.

CHAPTER TWO

Pathology of the Immune Response

The immune response is a finely balanced system which, when triggered by foreign antigen, should react to quickly and efficiently clear the foreign substance (Fig. 2.1). Once the foreign antigens have been removed, homeostatic control mechanisms should modulate the system to curtail any unnecessary response. The immune system, in addition, retains memory of these particular foreign antigens and the ability to respond to them even more quickly the second time around. Although the immune response is a marvelously complex system which usually serves to protect us, derangements of this system can lead to severe, sometimes life-threatening disease. In this chapter, we consider the pathology of the immune system, first summarizing immunodeficiency disorders and then discussing immune reactivity, which results in injury to the host or immunologically mediated diseases.

IMMUNODEFICIENCY DISEASES

As noted in Chapter 1, host defense against assault by microbial pathogens can be classified as nonspecific (especially phagocytosis and killing) and specific (humoral and cell-mediated) responses. Congenital deficiencies of any of the cellular functions required for these responses can lead to increased susceptibility to pathogens as well as organisms which are not usually pathogenic for normal individuals. Patients with selective immune deficiencies have been "experiments of nature" and have taught us much about the functions of the immune response and the

specific requirements for resistance to certain organisms. Deficiencies of phagocytosis, humoral immunity, cellular immunity, and complement have been described in man.[1] In addition, acquired immunodeficiencies, usually of a more generalized nature, have been associated with cancer and immunosuppressive therapies.

Intrinsic deficiencies of phagocytic cells are caused by deficiencies of the enzymes which are normally necessary for the killing of ingested bacteria. There are several deficiencies of phagocytic cell function and each is associated with a different enzyme dysfunction. In general, these patients are usually very susceptible to bacterial infections but are able to deal adequately with viral and protozoal infections. For example, in Chediak-Higashi disease, lysosomes are structurally and functionally abnormal so that these patients are susceptible to pyogenic bacteria.

Deficiencies of humoral immunity range from the complete absence of all immunoglobulins to the selective deficiency of a single immunoglobulin class (most commonly IgA). Likewise, the associated susceptibility to pyogenic bacterial infections also varies from mild to severe, depending on the immunoglobulin deficiency. In Bruton's congenital agammaglobulinemia, patients are susceptible to infections with pyogenic bacteria and *Pneumocystis carinii*. In addition, patients with marked immunoglobulin deficiency have been found to demonstrate an increased susceptibility to certain viral infections. Patients with humoral immune deficiencies respond well

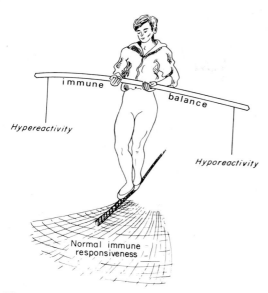

immune balance

Hyperreactivity

Hyporeactivity

Normal immune responsiveness

Figure 2.1 The immune response is a finely balanced system. The lack of sufficient response or hyporeactivity might allow infection to overwhelm the host, while hyperreactivity might result in immunologically mediated disease which could also be deleterious.

to treatment with gammaglobulin, which supplies specific antibodies against pathogens they are likely to encounter.

Disorders of cell-mediated immunity (T-cell) without a humoral immunodeficiency are rare. Since cooperation between T-cells and B-cells is required for antibody production to most antigens, lack of T-cell function usually results in a lack of the capacity to make specific antibodies. Since the thymus is necessary for differentiation of cells required for the cell-mediated immune response, congenital aplasia of the organ, or DiGeorge syndrome, results in severe deficiency of the cell-mediated immune response. Patients with T-cell deficiencies are usually susceptible to a variety of microbial organisms including viral, fungal, and protozoal infections.

A number of congenital deficiencies of both humoral and cell-mediated immunity have been described. These disorders range in severity from the relatively mild diseases of unknown etiology to the severe deficiencies associated with defects of the stem cells which differentiate into

T-cells, B-cells, or macrophages. Patients with severe combined immunodeficiency (Swiss-type) have a deficiency of stem cells and are highly susceptible to pathogenic and nonpathogenic microbial organisms and must be transplanted with competent, syngeneic stem cells (from bone marrow) in order to be able to survive normally in the sea of organisms that surrounds us. Ataxia telangiectasia is associated with depressions of both cell-mediated immunity and humoral immunity (deficiencies of IgA and IgE). Patients with the Wiskott-Aldrich syndrome (eczema, thrombocytopenia, recurrent infections) also display deficiencies in both cellular and humoral immunity that may be the result of a defect in macrophage presentation of antigen.

A variety of complement deficiencies have been described, some of which have been associated with greater than normal susceptibility to bacterial infections.[2] A deficiency of C1 inhibitor is associated with hereditary angioneurotic edema which is characterized by intermittent episodes of swelling of the skin and upper respiratory and gastrointestinal tracts. In these patients, uninhibited cleavage of C4 and C2 by C1 results in a marked reduction in serum levels of these complement components and increased vascular permeability mediated by a fragment of C2. The most common inherited complement deficiency is a deficiency of C2. This complement deficiency is associated with systemic lupus erythematosus. A deficiency of C3 is associated with increased susceptibility to severe, life-threatening pyogenic infections. C3-deficient serum does not support complement-mediated functions such as bactericidal activity, chemotaxis, and immune adherence. A deficiency of C3b inactivator results in spontaneous activation of the alternative complement pathway with resultant low levels of C3 and factor B. Many complement-mediated functions are severely depressed or absent, and these patients have a marked increase in susceptibility to bacterial infections. Patients with homozygous deficiencies of C5, C6, C7, and C8 also have increased susceptibility to infection, particularly with *Neisseria*. In Leiner's disease or C5 dysfunction syndrome there is an abnormality of C5 function that is associated with severe dermatitis, diarrhea, recurrent infections, and marked wasting. C9 deficiency does not seem to adversely affect health.

A number of diseases have been associated with secondary immunodeficiency. These deficiencies are usually transient and associated with the active phase of the primary disease. As examples, tuberculosis, sarcoidosis, and leprosy induce anergy. The immunodeficiency that is often associated with cancer is either induced by the malignant cells through suppressor cells which suppress normal responses or develops because of the cytotoxic drugs used to treat cancer and their suppressive effect on the immune system. The importance of secondary immunodeficiencies is that they usually affect phagocytic cells and cell-mediated immunity and cause an increased susceptibility to microbial pathogens as well as to organisms which are not normally pathogenic.

IMMUNOLOGICALLY MEDIATED DISEASES

Damage which results from the response of one's own immune system can be considered in two somewhat distinct categories. Immunologically mediated disease may be the result of a direct immune response against one's own tissue antigens. Such autoimmune diseases appear to result from the breakdown of the normal tolerance to "self" tissue antigens that may or may not be triggered by an infectious agent. The other form of immunologically mediated disease can be thought of more as injury incidental to an immune response against foreign antigens (Fig. 2.2). These are thought of as hypersensitivity reactions since the response, and damage caused by it, appear to be greatly exaggerated.

Autoimmune Diseases

If one of the main requirements of the immune response is to recognize foreign substances and eliminate them, a direct corollary of this is that the immune response must be able to recognize self-

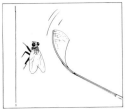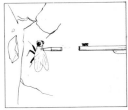

APPROPRIATE RESPONSE   HYPERSENSITIVITY
                                 (Allergic Response)

Figure 2.2 An appropriate immune response is depicted as using a fly swatter to eliminate the fly. An appropriate immune response eliminates the foreign substance with minimal damage to the host. Conversely, hypersensitivity might be considered a much greater response to an antigen than is necessary. Thus, the cartoon showing a fly being killed by a rifle. The incidental damage to the wall is far more than what was necessary.

antigens and not respond and attempt to eliminate them. In other words, a form of self-tolerance must be enacted so that the immune response does not turn against the host. Breakdown of this self-tolerance results in autoimmune diseases such as rheumatoid arthritis and systemic lupus erythematosus. Autoimmune disease implies that tissue injury is caused by an immunological reaction of the organism against its own tissues.[3] Autoimmunity on the other hand refers merely to the presence of antibody or lymphocytes that react with self-antigens but does not necessarily imply pathogenic significance. In this case, self-reactivity may be a consequence of a pathological process rather than the cause of it.

A breakdown of self-tolerance may result from alterations in the immunogenicity and availability of self-antigens. These alterations may be important in organ-specific autoimmune diseases such as autoimmune thyroiditis, pemphigus vulgaris, autoimmune hemolytic anemia, idiopathic thrombocytopenic purpura, myasthenia gravis, and sympathetic ophthalmia. One possibility is that unaltered antigenic material might be released from sites that are normally excluded from immune surveillance. This may apply to lens proteins which do not usually enter the general circulation. This mechanism may have only limited importance, however, since many antigens that were originally thought to be hidden from the immune system, such as thyroglobulin, have been shown to be normally present in the circulation. A second mechanism for the development of autoimmunity involves exposure of the organism to exogenous antigens that stimulate the production of antibody or antigen-stimulated lymphocytes, which in turn cross-react with self-antigens. Autoimmune responses may also result from alterations of self-antigens that render them immunogenic. Mechanisms for altering self-antigens include drugs, viral infections, or denaturation as a result of inflammation.

Systemic autoimmune disease with their diversity of autoreactivity might result from a more general activation of the immune system rather than from alterations in individual self-antigens. Examples of systemic autoimmune diseases include systemic lupus erythematosus and Sjögren's syndrome. Autoimmunity in such diseases may result from polyclonal B-cell activation with the formation of multiple autoantibodies or diffuse activation of helper T-cell activity. On the other hand, autoimmunity may not result from overstimulation of the immune system but rather from a deficiency of immunoregulatory mechanisms. Clinical experience in combination with studies of animal models of autoimmune diseases suggest that self-tolerance is probably due to an active suppressor cell response which inhibits the response against self-antigens and that human and animal autoimmune diseases result from defects in the generation and expression of suppressor T-cell activity.[4] The pathogenesis of autoimmune disorders may then be due to a failure of suppressor cell function. Lack of suppressor cell function probably leads to an imbalance in the immune response whereby helper T-cells are allowed to promote responses to self as well as to foreign antigens.

Autoimmune diseases may in the final analysis result from an interplay of many factors and may not be explained by a single underlying mechanism. A number of abnormalities may interact to induce the complete syndrome. Important determinants in the induction of autoimmunity include age, sex, genetic background, exposure to infectious agents, and environmental contacts.

Hypersensitivity Reactions

Most commonly, hypersensitivity or allergic reactions are classified on a clinical basis as immediate or delayed reactions. This classification is based simply on the time required for the reaction to appear after challenge with antigen. However, recent laboratory advances in understanding the cellular basis of immune reactions have allowed a more accurate description of hypersensitivity reactions based on a more complete understanding of the mechanisms involved. Gell and Coombs have classified the reactions resulting in tissue damage into four categories. Types I, II, and III depend on the interaction of antigen and humoral antibody and tend to present clinically as "immediate" type reactions, while Type IV reactions are mediated by the cell-mediated immune arm of the immune response and have a delayed course of development.[5] Although based on the time course of development of the reactions, this classification also reflects the different mechanisms which can be involved. As will be seen below, there is some overlapping between types of reactions, and during any given disease several types of reactions may occur simultaneously. However, this classification is extremely useful for understanding the immune mechanisms that result in tissue injury.

TYPE I - ANAPHYLACTIC HYPERSENSITIVITY

Anaphylactic reactions are the most immediate of the hypersensitivity reactions. Type I reactions are caused by the release of pharmacologically active substances by basophils and mast cells subsequent to the reaction between antigen and specific antibody adsorbed to the cell membrane (Fig. 2.3). Exposure to antigens such as drugs, pollen, or microbes may result in an IgE antibody, which binds through the Fc receptor to basophils or mast cells that are capable of releasing the various mediators of these reactions. Re-exposure to the sensitizing antigen, even in very small

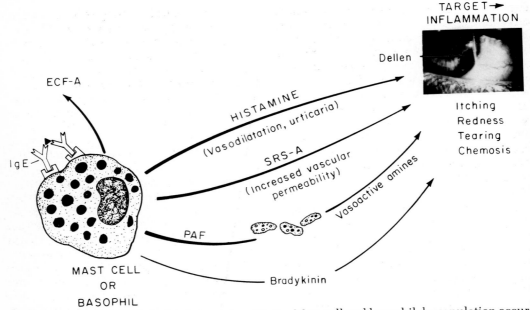

Figure 2.3 Type I - anaphylactic hypersensitivity. Mast cell and basophil degranulation occurs following the interaction of allergen with bound homocytotropic (reaginic) IgE antibody. Several pharmacological mediators are released which result in the symptoms of immediate type allergy. If the eye is the target of the localized reaction, the symptoms are itching, redness, tearing, and chemosis.

amounts, can trigger release of the active substances. Patients who exhibit such reactions to antigens are said to be allergic. Reagenic (IgE) antibodies are usually responsible for these reactions and are found in much higher concentrations in patients with a history of allergy or asthma.

Reactions following re-exposure to allergen occur very rapidly, often within a few minutes, and can be localized or systemic. A skin test with allergen produces a typical wheal and flare. Administration of an allergen in the eye is followed promptly by itching, tearing, redness, and chemosis. Desensitization following the repeated injection of minute quantities of allergen is often successful. This treatment is thought to work either by inducing the formation of blocking antibody, which combines readily and specifically with the antigen and neutralizes it, or by exhaustively degranulating the mediator cells.

The mediators released from mast cells and basophils are responsible for the pathophysiological changes in allergic disease. They can be divided into primary and secondary mediators, with secondary mediators being released indirectly as a consequence of the primary immune events. There are at least five mediators of inflammation released by mast cells and basophils including histamine, slow-reacting substance of anaphylaxis (SRS-A), platelet activating factor (PAF), basophil kallikrein of anaphylaxis (BK-A), and eosinophilic chemotactic factor of anaphylaxis (ECF-A) (Fig. 2.3). The release of histamine results in increased vascular permeability, vasodilation, and one of the most characteristic symptoms of allergy, itching. The biological activities of SRS-A are similar to histamine except that they develop slowly and last longer. PAF induces platelet aggregation which then becomes another source of histamine. BK-A eventually results in the production of secondary mediators such as kinins which further increase vascular permeability. ECF-A attracts eosinophils to the site of mast cell degranulation, where they neutralize the effects of some of the released mediators by producing the following chemicals: histaminase, arylsulfatase B, and phospholipase D, which destroy histamine, SRS-A, and PAF, respectively. Therefore, eosinophils are often found in high concentration at the site of allergic reactions, probably to modulate the effects of the mediators released by the mast cells. Eosinophils may also be able to ingest and destroy whole mast cell granules before their mediator contents escape to the tissue (Fig. 2.4).

The secondary mediators are released as a consequence of the primary immune response and include such chemicals as serotonin, bradykinin, and some of the prostaglandins. Serotonin has been found to have a role in anaphylaxis in animals but not man. Bradykinin results from the action of BK-A on serum kininogen. In humans, it causes a slow, sustained contraction of smooth muscles, increased permeability, increased secretions of mucous glands, and stimulation of pain fibers. Prostaglandins are a family of biologically, highly active lipids which are present in most tissues and are released upon damage to that tissue. Physiologically, they result in more inflammation by increasing capillary permeability and smooth muscle contraction. Injury due to the primary inflammatory response results in the release of secondary mediators that increase the inflammatory response. The inflammatory response may thus feed on itself to produce a vicious cycle.

The release of the various mediators by mast cells and basophils is at least partly under the control of the autonomic nervous system. The latter exerts its influence through the "second messenger" system (Fig. 2.5). Briefly, cholinergic or parasympathetic stimulation of guanylate cyclase, a cell membrane enzyme, causes an increase in the intracellular level of cyclic GMP. This is translated by the cell directly into an increase in the release of the mediators of inflammation. Conversely, adrenergic or sympathetic stimulation of another cell membrane enzyme, adenylate cyclase, results in the increase of intracellular levels of cyclic AMP and a concomitant decrease in the release of mediators. Because of their control over the release of effector molecules by mediator cells, these systems offer greater potential for treatment of anaphylactic reactions. Clearly, drugs which result in the increase of intracellular cyclic AMP should decrease mediator release and thereby decrease the symptoms of the reactions caused by the mediators.

TYPE II - ANTIBODY-DEPENDENT CYTOTOXIC HYPERSENSITIVITY

Immunological injury may also occur as a result of antibodies directed against

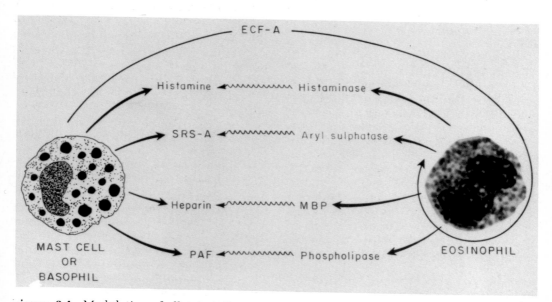

Figure 2.4 Modulation of allergic inflammation by the eosinophil. Eosinophilic chemotactic factor of anaphylaxis (ECF-A) released by the mast cell or basophil attracts eosinophils to the site of mast cells, where they neutralize the effects of some of the released mediators.

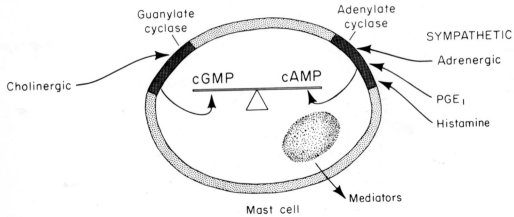

Figure 2.5 Modulation of mediator release by cyclic nucleotides. Second messenger system. Cholinergic stimulation of guanylate cyclase results in the increase of intracellular concentrations of cyclic GMP (cGMP), which augments release of mediators of immediate hypersensitivity. Adrenergic stimulation of adenylate cyclase augments cellular cyclic AMP (cAMP) and reduces mediator release. Cyclic AMP and cyclic GMP are the intracellular messengers of these intercellular messages. Their balance dictates the level of mediator release, and drugs which modulate their concentration effectively modulate mediator release and thus hypersensitivity reactions.

structural antigens on a cell surface or antigens which have adhered to a cell surface. After combination of the antibody with the antigen at the cell surface, damage to the cell can be accomplished by any of three mechanisms (Fig. 2.6). First, the antibody with or without complement may induce the phagocytosis of the cell by macrophages which have Fc receptors for the Fc portion of antibody and C3b receptors for this fragment of complement. Second, the antibody on the cell surface might activate complement which, if the cascade is completed, would result in lysis of the cell. Third, the antibody on the cell surface might provide the Fc component required for the binding of killer cells which would then lyse the target cell. Red blood cell lysis is the most important clinical example involving Type II reactions. Transfusions with allogeneic cells can result in antibodies which cause lysis of the red blood cells. Similarly, alteration of red cell antigens by viruses or drugs can induce antibodies which lyse red blood cells.

TYPE III - IMMUNE COMPLEX MEDIATED HYPERSENSITIVITY

Soluble antigen can combine with antibody to form antigen-antibody complexes which localize in tissue and induce an inflammatory response. The immune complexes bind complement, which results in the release of complement components chemotactic for leukocytes. Platelets are damaged and release vasoactive amines which cause increased vascular permeability. Antigen-antibody complexes are then localized in blood vessel walls where they fix complement and release chemotactic factors which cause the infiltration of the region with polymorphonuclear leukocytes (PMNs). The PMNs ingest the immune complexes and release lysosomal enzymes which damage adjacent cells and tissues.

If immune complexes are confined to the site of antigen introduction or local lymphoid tissue, they have only minor immunopathological consequences. However, circulating complexes appear to have a predisposition for basement membranes (Fig. 2.7). These complexes thus are deposited on basement membranes underlying the cells that line blood vessels as well as the basement membranes of other tissues. In the kidneys the complexes get caught in the filtration slits in the basement membranes of glomerular capillaries where the fluid passes through, thus destroying filtering integrity.

The outcome of the formation of immune complexes in vivo depends on the amount of immune complexes as well as on the relative proportions of antibody to antigen in the complexes. Large amounts of immune complexes result in their phagocytosis and clearance, while small amounts are readily passed out. Intermediate amounts can be trapped in tissues and cause immune complex disease. In addition, when in antibody excess, insoluble complexes are formed which are rapidly precipitated and tend to localize, resulting in tissue damage, e.g., Arthus reaction. When in antigen excess, soluble complexes are formed which may cause systemic reactions with deposition in the kidneys, joints and skin, e.g., serum sickness.

Recurrent or continuous immune complex disease occurs when the inducing antigens are endogenous, as in collagen disease, or are produced by infectious organisms which cannot be eliminated. Such conditions result in the continuous formation of immune complexes and their deposition on basement membranes. Although in some immune complex diseases the antigen is unknown, the disease can be diagnosed by the presence of the immune complexes (including immunoglobulin and complement) on basement membranes of skin or kidneys.

Immune complexes may deposit in systemic blood vessels to cause necrotizing vasculitis or deposit in joints to cause arthritis. Rheumatoid arthritis is an example of an immune complex disease in which the antigen appears to be an abnormal IgG molecule which complexes with Rheumatoid factor, a circulating IgM immunoglobulin which binds the IgG

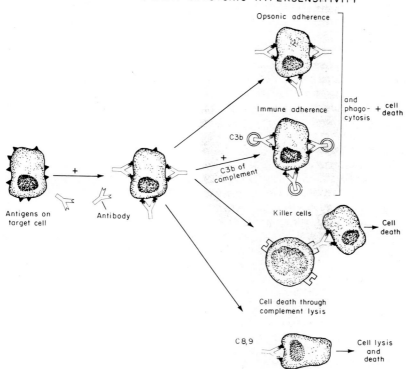

TYPE II ANTIBODY-DEPENDENT CYTOTOXIC HYPERSENSITIVITY

Figure 2.6 Type II - antibody-dependent cytotoxic hypersensitivity. Antibody directed against cell-surface antigens (adsorbed foreign antigens, changed self, or allogeneic cell) results in cell death. 1) Increased phagocytosis through opsonic adherence or immune adherence; 2) killer cells bind to bound antibody through Fc receptor and lyse target cell; 3) complement-dependent lysis (entire cascade needed).

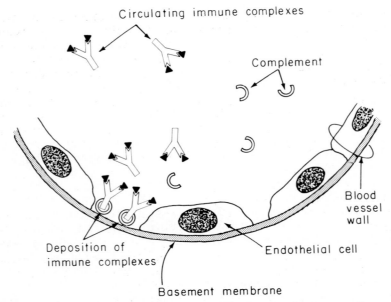

Figure 2.7 Immune complex disease. Antigen-antibody complexes may form and become lodged on the basement membrane. The immune complexes activate complement, which helps initiate an inflammatory response. Usually this results in elimination of the complexes. However, if the antigen is reintroduced or chronically produced, immune complex disease ensues.

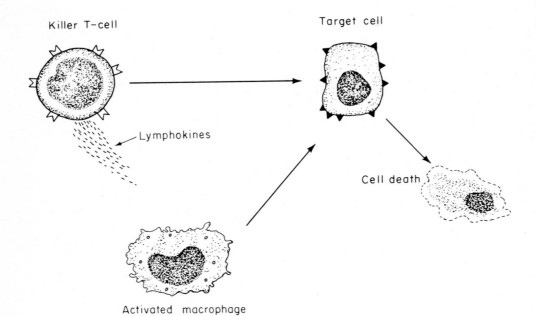

Figure 2.8 Type IV - cell-mediated (delayed) hypersensitivity. When sensitive T-cells are re-exposed to an antigen, they respond by making lymphokines which attract and activate macrophages, polymorphonuclear leukocytes, and other cells. These cells can nonspecifically cause damage to innocent bystander cells. The T-cells can also become cytotoxic and kill and target cells bearing the foreign antigen.

molecule. In the eye, scleral deposits of these immune complexes result in scleritis.

TYPE IV - CELL-MEDIATED HYPERSENSITIVITY

Cell-mediated immune responses are the result of an interaction between previously sensitized T-lymphocytes and specific antigen and are mediated by the release of lymphokines and by cytotoxicity (Fig. 2.8). The classical lesion associated with this response is the delayed skin reaction which requires 24–48 hours to develop and which demonstrates a characteristic mononuclear cell infiltrate. The lymphokines produced by the T-cells have their effects on a variety of cells including lymphocytes, PMNs, and macrophages. These lymphokines act to attract these cell populations to the site of the response, to make them divide, and to activate them to carry out certain functions at an increased rate. While these responses are usually beneficial since they are required for the elimination of certain intracellular bacterial pathogens, it is clear that the activated cells in these lesions can nonspecifically cause the death of cells other than those expressing the initial sensitizing antigen.

Cell-mediated immune hypersensitivity differs from the other types in that antibody does not appear to play a role and histamine is not involved. This delayed hypersensitivity is an important mechanism in many chronic ocular inflammatory diseases and contact allergies due to drugs, chemicals, and cosmetics. The chronic granulomatous diseases of infectious and noninfectious origin represent examples of cell-mediated immune hyperreactivity. These include sarcoidosis, sympathetic ophthalmia, tuberculosis, leprosy, syphilis, toxoplasmosis, and simple chalazia.

Granuloma formation results from the failure of phagocytic cells to eliminate microorganisms or other toxic products or antigens. This leads to encapsulation of the inciting agent into walled-off pockets. In tuberculosis, a good example of this phenomenon, activated macrophages engulf but fail to destroy the tubercle bacillus. A prolonged local inflammatory reaction results from replication of these organisms inside the activated macrophage. The combination of activated macrophages and surrounding inflammatory cells develop into a nodule which is identifiable histologically as a granuloma. As a granuloma enlarges, there is a proliferation of fibrous tissue at the outer margin and necrosis at the center.

SUMMARY

Diseases of the immune system can be divided into immunodeficiency diseases and immunologically mediated diseases. Immunodeficiency can result from an inborn error of metabolism which affects a specific cell required for immune response or can be secondary to immunosuppression caused by therapies or certain diseases. Immunologically mediated diseases result from the loss of self-tolerance or as a side-effect of an immune response against foreign antigen. The latter are termed hypersensitivity reactions and have been classified as four types which depend on the mechanisms involved.

REFERENCES

1. Soothill, J.F. Immunity deficiency states. In Clinical Aspects of Immunology, edited by Gell, P.G.H., Coombs, R.R.A., and Lachmann, P.J., third edition. Blackwell, Oxford, 1975, pp. 649–687.
2. Colten, H.R., Alper, C.A., Rosen, F.S. Genetics and biosynthesis of complement proteins. N. Engl. J. Med. 304:653–656, 1981.
3. Lipsky, P.E. Systemic autoimmune disease. Proceedings of Immunology of the eye. Workshop II, edited by Helmsen, R.J., Suran, A., Gery, I., and Nussenblatt, R.B. Immunology Abstr. (Suppl.) pp. 129–143, 1981.
4. Goodwin, J.S., Williams, R.C. Suppressor cells—A recent conceptual epidemic. J. Clin. Lab. Immunol. 2:89–91, 1979.
5. Coombs, R.R.A., Gell, P.G.H. Classification of allergic reactions responsible for clinical hypersensitivity and disease. In Clinical Aspects of Immunology, edited by Gell, P.G.H., Coombs, R.R.A., and Lachmann, P.J., third edition. Blackwell, Oxford, 1975, pp. 761–781.

CHAPTER THREE

Principles of Treatment

Modification of the immune response has been an active pursuit since before the time when immunity was found to be due to humoral or cellular factors. Basically, the hope has always been to be able to potentiate the immune response against invading pathogens and tumors or to be able to diminish immune responses which are deleterious to the host and transplanted organs. Augmentation of immunity has included such diverse approaches as vaccination, toxoid injections, passive transfer of immune serum, and the use of a host of natural and synthetic agents which have been shown to augment one aspect or another of the immune response and which have been termed immunopotentiators. Immunosuppression has also been approached in many different ways, e.g., specific antisera, cytotoxic drugs, or irradiation. In addition, management of allergic or hypersensitivity reactions can take advantage of our recently acquired understanding of the pathogenesis of the inflammatory reactions. In this chapter we will discuss the ways in which the immune response can be modified to 1) stimulate the normal immune response, 2) suppress the normal immune response, and 3) treat allergic diseases.

IMMUNOPOTENTIATION

Although the use of vaccines, toxoids and passive transfer of immunity with serum antibodies could all be considered to be immunopotentiation, the definition to be used here will include only those agents which are capable of enhancing the rate of development of an immune response, increasing the intensity of the response, or inducing a response with an otherwise nonimmunogenic substance. Using this definition, most of the immunopotentiators used in man are classified as adjuvants. For the purposes of this discussion, we will limit ourselves to consideration of the most commonly studied agents. It is of more than passing interest that several new immunopotentiators have recently been described which show great potential.

Bacillus Calmette-Guérin

Bacillus Calmette-Guérin (BCG) is a strain of *Mycobacterium bovis* which has been attenuated by repeated passage in culture medium enriched with beef bile. This agent was first developed for vaccination against tuberculosis, although its effectiveness has never been fully proven. Of late, it has been used as an immunopotentiator, especially in patients with cancer. It is thought to work by stimulating the reticuloendothelial system (RES) probably secondary to a cell-mediated (T-cell) immune response.[1] Since stimulation of the RES and the cell mediated immune response are thought to play an important role in defense against cancer and certain intracellular pathogens, it seemed logical to try to augment these responses with BCG.

Animal studies have clearly shown that BCG can delay the appearance, decrease the incidence, inhibit the development, and induce regression of experimentally induced tumors. In addition, BCG has been shown to augment resistance to certain bacterial and viral infections. Studies with BCG in man have been somewhat encouraging in patients with certain kinds of tumors but discouraging in patients with recurrent herpesvirus infections. Even though some studies of BCG in human cancer have shown signs of benefit to the patient, the optimal treatment regimens have not been defined. Furthermore, rare case reports have suggested that the BCG enhanced rather than diminished tumor spread. Side effects occur often and can be severe.

Several agents similar to BCG have also been used as immunopotentiators. Methanol extract residue (MER) of BCG and purified protein derivative (PPD) are similar in action to BCG. In addition, studies with the smallest active component derived from BCG, N-acetyl-muramyl-L-alanine-D-isoglutamine, have demonstrated this to be a potent immunopotentiator. *Corynebacterium parvum* is another organism which has been used to enhance the immune response by activating macrophages.

This approach to tumor therapy is not new. Many years ago Coley's fluid (a vaccine of *Streptococcus erysipelatis* and *Bacillus prodigiosus*) was used for sarcoma therapy.

Levamisole

Levamisole is a synthetic compound developed as a veterinary antihelminthic drug. It has also been found to augment the immune response to certain antigens and to enhance T-cell response to mitogens. In animal studies, levamisole has been shown to augment host resistance to tumors, especially in conjunction with cytotoxic drug therapy. In man, levamisole has been shown to enhance delayed skin reactions to antigens and dinitrochlorobenzene (DNCB). Some studies have claimed success with levamisole in virus infections but the lack of proper trials leaves these observations unproven.[2]

A number of newly synthesized compounds have been shown to have the capacity to augment various aspects of the immune response. However, evidence of their efficacy in man has not been developed.

Transfer Factor

Transfer factor can be prepared by lyophilizing the dialyzable extract of immune leukocytes. This material, when reconstituted and inoculated into a nonimmune individual, transfers from an immune donor delayed hypersensitivity to a specific antigen. Transfer factor has been shown to have a small molecular weight and may be a nucleopeptide. Transfer factor does not appear to be a homogeneous substance and its mode of action is not clear. However, unlike many other biological agents transfer factor appears to cause no serious side effects and has been shown to be beneficial to patients with certain immunodeficiencies, bacterial infections, viral infections, and fungal infections.[3]

Interferon

There are two classes of interferon that can be distinguished immunologically: type I, or standard interferon, and type II or immune interferon. Type I interferon is produced by fibroblasts, epithelial cells, macrophages, or leukocytes and can be induced by viruses, nucleic acids, synthetic polynucleotides, and bacterial products. Type II interferon is a lymphokine that is produced by specifically sensitized lymphocytes interacting with antigen or antigen-antibody complexes. Interferons are known to have antiviral, antitumor, and immunomodulatory activities and also have the capability of enhancing natural killer cell and macrophage activity.

Interferon is produced by virus-infected cells and is capable of rendering uninfected cells resistant to infection. For the most part, viruses that infect the eye, such as herpes simplex, varicella-zoster, adenovirus, vaccinia and certain picornaviruses, are relatively poor inducers of interferon.[4] In addition, these viruses are not particularly sensitive to interferon, especially when high levels of viruses are present.

Interferon has been found in the sera of patients with various autoimmune diseases including systemic lupus erythematosus, rheumatoid arthritis, scleroderma and Sjögren's syndrome.[5] Since interferon alters immune responses, it is possible that it may contribute to certain immunological aberrations found in these diseases.

IMMUNOSUPPRESSION

As with immunopotentiation, immunosuppression can be induced by natural products as well as by synthetic agents. This discussion will be limited to cytotoxic drugs, corticosteroids, antilymphocyte serum, and irradiation. The capacity of the various treatment modalities to be immunosuppressive depends on three factors. First, the primary immune response is much easier to diminish than is a response after it has been established. This is because the primary response requires extensive proliferation, which makes cells of the immune response sensitive to the treatments. Second, the timing of the immunosuppressive drug is very important. Some of these drugs are effective only during certain portions of the cell proliferation cycle and thus must be given when the immune cells are at that point. Third, not all cells of the immune response are equally sensitive to the various treatments. Thus, the sensitivities of the various populations of cells will determine the effect of the treatment.

Cytotoxic Drugs

Cytotoxic drugs are designed to kill immunologically competent cells. These drugs are highly specific for DNA replication, kill proliferating cells in general, or kill proliferating and nonproliferating cells equally. Azathioprin, a purine analog, is an example of a drug which interferes with DNA synthesis and thus kills actively proliferating cells. It is one of the prime drugs used to inhibit graft rejection in renal transplant recipients and has been used to treat patients with autoimmune disorders. Methotrexate also acts to inhibit DNA synthesis and is used to treat patients with autoimmune diseases.

Cyclophosphamide is an alkylating agent which cross-links cellular DNA and causes the death of cells when they proliferate. It is highly immunosuppressive and has been found to be especially useful in patients with autoimmune disorders.

Since cytotoxic drugs usually are active against replicating cells, the other rapidly proliferating cells of the body can and often are affected similarly. These drugs are, therefore, highly toxic to bone marrow cells, to the cells of the gastrointestinal epithelium, and to the germinal cells of the gonads. Suppression of the bone marrow is probably the most important consideration since this results in marked susceptibility to pathogenic organisms as well as to otherwise nonpathogenic microbes. Of particular importance are infections with intracellular parasites. There are also indications that patients treated with immunosuppressive drugs are more susceptible to cancer. This is probably due to loss of immune surveillance as a result of the immunosuppression but may be due to the carcinogenic properties of some of these compounds.

Corticosteroids

Corticosteroids are the most widely used agents in the treatment of inflammatory and immunologically mediated disease. In man, corticosteroids do not mediate their immunosuppressive effects by killing cells. Rather, they appear to do so by affecting the functions of certain cell populations and their distribution. In discussing the mechanism of action of corticosteroids, it is difficult to clearly separate anti-inflammatory from immunosuppressive effects. The anti-inflammatory effects of corticosteroids are nonspecific with regard to the causes of disease processes and will inhibit the inflammatory reaction to nearly any type of stimulus. The effects of corticosteroids are numerous[6,7] and include the following:

1. Inhibition of the increased capillary permeability induced by acute inflammation, so that there is less leakage of fluid, proteins and inflammatory cells into an inflammatory site.
2. Stabilization of lysosomes which contain enzymes that cause tissue damage.
3. Lymphocytopenia. In man, T-lymphocytes are more susceptible to the effects of corticosteroids than B-lymphocytes. Thus, antibody production is rarely reduced significantly except with very large doses of corticosteroids, whereas cell-mediated immunity is modified at lower corticosteroid concentrations.
4. Interference with phagocytosis and

digestion of antigen by macrophages.

5. Eosinopenia.
6. Inhibition of migration of macrophage and polymorphonuclear leukocytes into inflamed areas by inhibiting their adherence to the capillary endothelium and subsequent passage through the capillary wall.
7. Inhibition of lymphocyte stimulation and transformation to mitogens.
8. Suppression of immediate hypersensitivity reactions by increasing the levels of adenyl cyclase and cyclic AMP, thereby diminishing the release of vasoactive amines.
9. Inhibition of prostaglandin synthesis.

As with the cytotoxic drugs, the side effects of prolonged treatment with corticosteroids can be a cause of great morbidity.

Antilymphocyte Serum

In recent years, the use of antilymphocyte serum (ALS) in the suppression of renal graft rejection has gained great popularity. ALS is a highly effective immunosuppressant which has been shown to suppress both cell-mediated and humoral immunity by depletion of certain lymphocyte populations. Although used as treatment for certain autoimmune reactions, ALS has been found to be most useful in the treatment of graft rejection. In addition to the usual side effect of increased susceptibility to infection, this immunosuppressive treatment has also been associated with serum sickness.

X-ray Irradiation

X-ray irradiation has also been shown to be immunosuppressive and has been used clinically to immunosuppress patients prior to bone marrow transplantation. Irradiation causes the death of most lymphocytes and other dividing cells. The side effects are thus numerous and serious.

Newer Approaches

As noted in Chapter 1, an understanding of the mechanisms which are responsible for immunological homeostasis is now being developed. It is clear that the immune system generates highly specific suppressor molecules which control the host's response to self and certain foreign antigens. It is our belief that in the years ahead these suppressor molecules will be made in culture and supplied to individuals lacking them. These should mediate highly specific suppression without subjecting the host to undue risks of infection or malignancy.

MANAGEMENT OF THE ALLERGIC RESPONSE

Prerequisites for the successful management of allergic reactions in general and of the eye in particular are 1) the recognition that an allergy is present; 2) the proper classification of the allergic mechanism involved; and 3) the discovery, if possible, of the sensitizing substance. On many occasions, because ocular allergies often resemble inflammations of nonallergic origin, such as bacterial and viral infections or reactions to direct primary irritants, allergy is not recognized when it is present or is erroneously diagnosed when it does not exist. Therefore, unless each case is properly evaluated, serious problems in the management of these patients may arise, problems that modern day therapy may aggravate rather than resolve.

The therapeutic regime in allergy of the eyes should be as follows.

Avoidance

The ideal treatment of allergy is to find the cause and avoid the antigen. If the cause cannot be eliminated, major reliance should be placed on nonspecific measures and drugs. Desensitization is reserved for special instances. An important principle, especially in contact allergies, is the avoidance of any medication in the treatment which may arouse new sensitivities in highly sensitized tissues not likely to be allergic to these drugs at other times.

Desensitization

Desensitization is employed with success in some patients with asthma and hay fever and also in situations where a chronic microbiallergic reaction to staphylococci or staphylococcus exotoxin occurs in the outer eye. Other vaccines were used with occasional success in uveitis before the availability of corticosteroids. Hyposensitization or desensitization required periodic intradermal or subcutaneous injections of the allergen in increasing doses, which cause a reduction of the level of circulating IgE. There is usually a rise in allergen specific blocking IgG that may compete with IgE for the allergen. Desensitization may also generate suppressor cells with histamine receptors that specifically suppress a proliferative response to the antigen and may be partly responsible for the efficacy of this therapy.[8]

Pharmacological Approach

Virtually every step in the pathogenesis of an allergic reaction can be used as a target for the pharmacologic suppression of these reactions (Fig. 3.1).

CYCLIC AMP

As noted earlier (Chapter 2), the functions of mediator cells are influenced by the autonomic nervous system. Agents which result in an increase in cyclic AMP cause a reduction in the release of vasoactive amines while agents which depress the intracellular concentration of cyclic AMP augment mediator release. Because of this, agents which cause an increase in

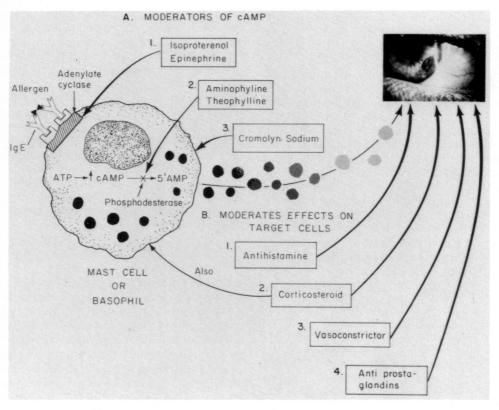

Figure 3.1 Composite diagram and photograph showing pharmacological manipulation of both the release of mediators and the control of effects they have on target cells of the eye. *A*, moderators of cyclic AMP (cAMP). Drugs that increase intracellular levels of cyclic AMP and therefore decrease mediator release include: 1) adrenergic compounds such as isoproterenol and epinephrine which stimulate adenylate cyclase; 2) aminophylline and theophylline, which inhibit phosphodiesterase, the enzyme which breaks down cyclic AMP; 3) cromolyn sodium, which is thought to prevent the degranulation of mast cells by stabilizing lysosomal membranes. *B*, drugs that moderate the effects of released mediators on target cells include: 1) antihistamines; 2) corticosteroids; 3) vasoconstrictors; 4) prostaglandin inhibitors.

intracellular cyclic AMP, either by greater production through the enzyme adenyl cyclase (e.g., isoproterenol and epinephrine) or by preventing the breakdown of intracellular cyclic AMP through inhibition of the enzyme phosphodiesterase (e.g., aminophylline), cause less mediator release and therefore a reduction in the allergic reaction.

INHIBITION OF DEGRANULATION

Cromolyn sodium acts to stabilize lysosomal membranes and thus prevent the release of mediators. Corticosteroids may also act in this manner.

MODERATORS OF EFFECTS ON TARGET CELLS

Another level at which pharmacological intervention can be attempted is inhibition of the effects of the released mediators.

Antihistamines. The basis of antihistamine therapy is, first, histamine plays a prominent part in anaphylaxis and in certain other forms of allergy, and second, antihistaminics nullify histamine action by combining with the target cell at the histamine receptor, preventing the absorption of histamine by these cells and, thus, the resultant allergic reaction.

Histamine levels have been measured in normal tears and have been found to be elevated in vernal conjunctivitis but not hay fever conjunctivitis.[9] The human ocular surface may contain both H_1- and H_2-receptors for histamine.[10] Although both ocular hyperemia and itching are induced by histamine, an H_1-agonist produces itching as the primary effect with no mucous discharge or vasodilation, while an H_2-agonist produces dilation of episcleral, conjunctival, and perilimbal ciliary vessels but no sensation of itching, stinging, or burning. Antazoline, an H_1-antagonist, inhibits itching; cimetidine, an H_2-antagonist, blocks vasodilation.[10–12] The therapeutic value of topical antihistaminics is questionable, and for improved therapeutic value, topical antihistaminic preparations may need to contain both H_2-receptor and H_1-receptor antagonists.

If the oral use of antihistaminics is of value in patients suffering from seasonal hay fever, the conjunctivitis associated with this allergic response is often greatly alleviated, even if not completely eradicated. Systemically administered antihistamines, however, produce a variety of side effects including sedation, dizziness, nervousness, insomnia, muscular weakness, gastrointestinal disturbances, and dryness of the mouth.

Since histamine plays little or no demonstrable role in delayed hypersensitivity, one should not expect, nor does one find, antihistaminics to be of value in either contact or microbial allergies. As a side effect, antihistaminics frequently cause allergy, and they were discontinued in the ointment form because of such allergic reactions.

Corticosteroids. Corticosteroids increase levels of adenyl cyclase and cyclic cAMP, thereby reducing the release of vasoactive amines. They also potentiate the effects of β-adrenergic catecholamines. However, the abuse of the steroids has detracted from the great advantages these products offer. Their use in the eyes is not without danger.

Adverse effects from the local use of steroids for ocular allergies include allergic and irritative reactions, the triggering of infections with the virus of herpes simplex, the possibility of introducing bacterial infection by means of contaminated solutions, the diminishing of host resistance so that secondary bacterial and mycotic infections may arise, the occurrence of steroid glaucoma, and, in prolonged usage, the development of cataracts in some patients.

The widespread use of steroids in combination with antibacterial agents has inadvertently accentuated these dangers. Beguiled by the apparently logical basis for these combinations, as promoted by their manufacturers who cite their broad value against both bacterial infections and allergies, they are used with abandon, not so much by ophthalmologists, but by other physicians, often for long and disastrous periods of time. Since only ophthalmologists are equipped to recognize herpetic infections of the cornea, warnings against the use of these products for such viral infections, now common in the pharmaceutical literature provided, are without any real meaning.

Contamination of ophthalmic solutions

by pathologic bacteria as a cause of serious corneal infection was highlighted by the introduction of commercially prepared ophthalmic cortisone solutions. Due to lack of proper precautions, gross infection with *Pseudomonas aeruginosa* (*Bacillus pyocyaneus*) occurred. This led to Federal Drug Administration (FDA) regulations in 1953, first initiated by Theodore and by Theodore and Feinstein,[13, 14] requiring the sterile preparation of all commercial ophthalmic solutions.

Central corneal ulcers due to infections with many varieties of bacteria as well as so-called benign contaminant fungi have occurred due to the immunosuppressive action of corticosteroids, when used for prolonged periods for allergies, chronic herpetic corneal infections, and other types of corneal problems.

In regard to the prevention of steroid glaucoma and steroid cataract, the importance—especially in children and those in nursing homes—of regularly scheduled reexaminations deserves emphasis. Finally, a good general rule to follow when prescribing long-term steroid therapy is to warn the patient of possible complications, stressing the need for return visits.

Vasoconstrictors. Since the pathophysiology of some of the allergic reactions of the external eye involve an exudative response with vasodilation, vasoconstrictors can be useful in treating these problems. Topical vasoconstrictors such as epinephrine, ephedrine, phenylephrine, and naphazoline are highly effective in the relief of acute allergic conjunctivitis. Cold compresses are also excellent in giving temporary relief from itching and may act by causing vasoconstriction. In chronic atopic conjunctivitis, where there is less vasodilation and edema, less emphasis should be placed on vasoconstrictors.

Antiprostaglandins. Indomethacin and aspirin are of theoretical value in inhibiting the synthesis of prostaglandins which are released as a result of inflammation and the damage caused by it. However, since the role of prostaglandins in allergic reactions is very complex, it is possible that their inhibition will have countervailing results.

Cyclosporin A. Cyclosporin A is a peptide of fungal origin that has important suppressive effects on T-lymphocytes but only minimal suppressive effects on B-lymphocytes.[15] This immunosuppressive is now receiving widespread attention because it prolongs the survival of allografts. Hepatotoxicity and increased frequency of neoplasms have been reported with its use.

SUMMARY

A number of biologically active compounds are currently being used in the clinic to augment the immune response or to suppress it. Immunopotentiators are designed to augment the functions of certain cells of the immune response and augment resistance to infection or malignancy. Immunosuppression generally attempts to diminish the immune response by eliminating responsive cells or diminishing their capacities to participate in the response. The latter is used in treatment of immunologically mediated diseases. Treatment of allergic reactions depends on intervention at several levels to interrupt the chain of the hypersensitivity reaction.

REFERENCES

1. Mackaness, G.B., Lagrange, P.H., Ishibashi, T. The modifying effect of BCG on the immunological induction of T cells. J. Exp. Med. 139:1540, 1974.

2. Symoens, J., Brugman, J. Treatment of recurrent aphthous stomatitis and herpes with levamisole. Br. Med. J. 4:592, 1974.

3. Lawrence, H.S. Transfer factor. Adv. Immunol. 11:195, 1969.

4. Stanton, G.J., Langford, M.P., Weigent, D.A., Blalock, J.E., Baron, S. Amplifications of the interferon system that may influence infections of the eye. Proceedings of Immunology of the eye. Workshop III, edited by Suran, A., Gery, I., and Nussenblatt, R.B. Immunology Abstr. (Suppl.) pp. 443–457, 1981.

5. Hooks, J.J., Jordan, G.W., Moutsopoulos, H.M., Fauci, A.S., Abner, L.N. Autoimmune diseases and interferon. Proceedings of Immunology of the eye. Workshop II, edited by Helmsen, R.J., Suran, A., Gery, I., and Nussenblatt, R.B. Immunology Abstr. (Suppl.) pp. 207–216, 1981.

6. Leopold, I.H. Treatment of corneal diseases. Proceedings of Immunology of the eye. Workshop

II, edited by Helmsen, R.J., Suran, A., Gery, I., and Nussenblatt, R.B. Immunology Abstr. (Suppl.) pp. 103–119, 1981.

7. Melby, J.C. Systemic corticosteroid therapy: Pharmacology and endocrinologic considerations. Ann. Intern. Med. 81:505–512, 1974.

8. Rocklin, R.E., Sheffer, A.L., Greineder, D.K., Melmon, K.L. Generation of antigen-specific suppressor cells during allergy desensitization. N. Engl. J. Med. 302:1213–1218, 1980.

9. Allansmith, M.R., Baird, B.S., Higgenbothan, E.J., Abelson, M.B. Technical aspects of histamine determination in human tears. Am. J. Ophthalmol. 90:719–724, 1980.

10. Abelson, M.D., Udell, I.J.. H_2-receptors in the human ocular surface. Arch. Ophthalmol. 99:302–304, 1981.

11. Udell, I.J., Abelson, M.D. Animal and human ocular surface response to a topical nonimmune mast-cell degranulating agent (Compound 48/80). Am. J. Ophthalmol. 91:226–230, 1981.

12. Abelson, M.B., Allansmith, M.R., Friedlaender, M.H. Effects of topically applied ocular decongestant and antihistamine. Am. J. Ophthalmol. 90:254–257, 1980.

13. Theodore, F.H. Contamination of eye solutions. Am. J. Ophthalmol. 34:1764, 1951.

14. Theodore, F.H., Feinstein, R.R. Preparation and maintenance of sterile ophthalmic solutions. Report to A.M.A. Council on Pharmacy and Chemistry. JAMA 152:1631–1633, 1953.

15. Borel, J.F., Fewrer, C., Magnee, C. Effects of the new anti-lymphocyctic peptide cyclosporin A in animals. Immunology 32:1017–1025, 1972.

CHAPTER FOUR

The Conjunctiva

The conjunctiva may well be the best site in the body for the study of allergic reactions. Readily accessible mucous membrane juxtaposed to the adjacent thin and delicate skin of the eyelids provides an opportunity for all types of allergic reactions to occur to an extent and with a frequency not found elsewhere. While the nasal mucosa is often the site of explosive air-borne allergies, contact allergy is relatively rare. The reverse is true of the skin. Only in the conjunctiva are both of these forms of allergy, as well as reactions to microbial allergens, commonly encountered. Such allergic responses may result either from local exposure to excitants or as part of a generalized hypersensitivity.

Table 4.1 classifies the various types of conjunctival immune reactions that are encountered in clinical practice.

ATOPIC ALLERGIC CONJUNCTIVITIS

The term "atopic conjunctivitis" describes the conjunctival reaction occurring in systemic and localized anaphylactic reactions. A family history of allergy (atopy) is generally obtained. This is a clear-cut antigen-antibody response and should not be confused with the conjunctivitis occurring in so-called atopic dermatitis, which is by no means a clearly distinguished entity. As Table 4.1 indicates, atopic conjunctivitis is divided into acute and chronic varieties.

Acute Atopic Allergic Conjunctivitis

Acute atopic conjunctivitis is a type of hypersensitivity characterized by sudden or immediate hyperemia and edema. Marked chemosis of a glassy appearance occurs, usually associated with a watery discharge, although sometimes mucopurulent. It is the conjunctival prototype of the immediate type of allergic response and usually is caused by the air-borne group of allergens: pollens, animal danders and feathers, mold spores, dust, insects, and scents. The conjunctival reaction is similar to the general inflammatory edema which involves the upper respiratory tract.

Acute atopic allergic conjunctivitis is thought to be mediated by reaginic antibody (IgE) affixed to the surface of mast cells in the conjunctival stroma. Contact between the antigen and IgE triggers the release of those vasopermeability and leukotactic factors that result in the acute symptoms of allergy (Fig. 4.1).

A similar picture may occur in food allergies, such as allergies to eggs and milk, but in such cases the ocular reaction has only a minor role in a dramatic general systemic reaction.

As in the nasal symptoms of hay fever, the reaction may be so intense that a profuse mucopurulent discharge occurs. Itching and burning may be intolerable (Fig. 4.2). Eosinophils often occur in abundance in the secretions. Because vasodilation is a primary factor in this reaction, vasoconstrictors, like epinephrine, phenylephrine (Neo-Synephrine) hydrochloride, and naphazoline (Albalon, Vasocon, Privine) hydrochloride, help control the reaction which usually subsides once the excitant is removed. Sodium cromoglycate (Intal) may be of some help in certain patients with atopic conjunctivitis.

Skin tests of the intradermal type provoke an immediate wheal response in most patients with this type of hypersensitivity. Ophthalmic tests, by means of direct instillation of the suspected aller-

Table 4.1
Clinical Reactions of the Conjunctiva

1. *Atopic Conjunctivitis*
   Atopic (familial history of allergy); rarely, anaphylactic immediate allergic response (in a few minutes) after exposure. Positive intradermal wheal test in 15–30 minutes. Due to inhalants (pollens, dusts, fungi, animal epidermals) or foods.
   a. Acute atopic conjunctivitis:
      Major characteristics—itching, chemosis, eosinophilia
   b. Chronic atopic conjunctivitis:
      Major characteristics—itching, slight edema, eosinophilia
2. *Microbiallergic Conjunctivitis*
   Atopy not essential
   Delayed allergic response
   Delayed positive intradermal test (24–48 hours);
   Due to products of microorganisms: bacteria, fungi, parasites, possibly viruses
   Major characteristics—irritation, burning, some follicles
3. *Contact Dermatoconjunctivitis*
   Atopy not essential
   Delayed allergic responses (24–48 hours)
   Positive patch test in 1–5 days
   Contact allergy to locally applied drugs or chemicals: Major characteristics—papillary conjunctivitis, eyelid eczema
4. *Vernal Conjunctivitis*
5. *Conjunctivitis Associated with Atopic Dermatitis*
6. *Giant Papillary Conjunctivitis*
7. *Systemic Disorders with Conjunctival Involvement*
   a. Ocular cicatricial pemphigold
   b. Erythema multiforme (Stevens-Johnson syndrome)

gen in weak dilution, are generally not safe to perform in these patients. Severe and possibly permanent ocular damage may result. Because of chemosis, early epidemic keratoconjunctivitis may be confused with acute allergic conjunctivitis. The virus infection, however, is differentiated by the presence of preauricular lymphadenopathy and conjunctival follicles. On scrapings, mononuclear cells are found instead of eosinophils.

Chronic Atopic Allergic Conjunctivitis

In contradistinction to the often dramatic and generally severe reactions that occur in acute atopic conjunctivitis, the chronic form frequently shows little or no objective evidence of inflammation in comparison to the irritating subjective symptoms of itching, burning, photophobia, and dryness that are usually present. As a result, the patients often are considered psychoneurotic or else are thought to be suffering from chronic catarrhal conjunctivitis or dry eyes. Actually, since many cases of chronic conjunctivitis are found to be bacteriologically negative, it may be that a substantial number of such cases actually are misdiagnosed forms of chronic atopic conjunctivitis. In fact, even the ophthalmologist who is aware of the frequency of chronic atopic conjunctivitis and performs routine epithelial scrapings in conjunctivitis often is surprised to find numerous eosinophils in cases that clinically did not appear allergic.

The conjunctiva often appears rather pale. A minor degree of conjunctival edema may be suggested by the somewhat juicy appearance of the conjunctiva, especially in the lower fornix in its temporal portion. While the response is essentially papillary, follicles may appear in long-standing cases, especially where there is relatively little inflammatory reaction. In other patients, where a more subacute process occurs, there may be considerable injection, as well as slight chemosis. Corresponding to the grade of the reaction in general, there may be a slight watery discharge or a mucopurulent one. In either event, eosinophils are found on epithelial scrapings, always in diagnostic numbers, although less numerous than in acute atopic conjunctivitis. Chronic atopic conjunctivitis is often known as simple allergic conjunctivitis.

The diagnosis of chronic atopic conjunctivitis is often difficult because the condition may resemble other forms of chronic conjunctivitis, in particular microbiallergic conjunctivitis due to *Staphylococcus*. The conjunctivitis that occurs often does not permit any ready means of distinguishing between the two types, although there generally are slight differences. However, more important than the appearance of the conjunctiva itself are the history, the finding of eosinophils, and the response to certain types of therapy, such as local vasoconstrictors, steroids,

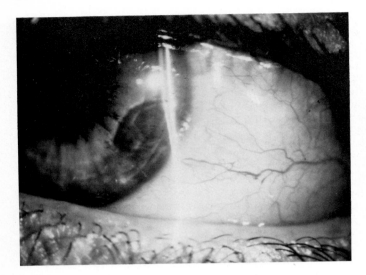

Figure 4.1 Acute atopic allergic conjunctivitis producing itching, tearing, redness and marked chemosis. The chemosis is severe enough to result in dellen formation of the peripheral cornea.

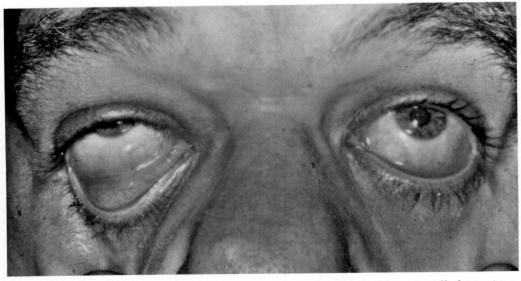

Figure 4.2 Ragweed sensitive patient in whom ragweed pollen had been instilled 22 minutes prior to photograph. (Reprinted with permission from Theodore, F.H., and Schlossman, A. Ocular Allergy. Williams & Wilkins, 1958.)

oral doses of antihistamine, and, if possible, elimination of the cause of the allergy. These clues provide the framework for differentiating chronic atopic conjunctivitis from other forms of chronic inflammation of the conjunctiva.

It must also be kept in mind that atopic patients are often compromised hosts. They have poor defenses against infectious agents, such as *Staphylococcus* and *Candida*. Secondary infection in the atopic individual must be considered in

one's approach to the diagnosis and treatment of the atopic individual.

MICROBIALLERGIC CONJUNCTIVITIS

The term "microbiallergic," coined by Theodore,[1] describes reactions resulting from microbial allergy. Many of the harmful effects that microorganisms can exert in the body are manifestations of allergy. Over and above the direct toxic nature of microbial infection, allergy or hypersensitivity may convert a harmless protein product of bacterial disintegration into a violent and destructive poison. Bacterial allergy, especially due to staphylococcal products, is of great importance in disease of the eyelid, conjunctiva, and cornea. Fungi and helminths also appear capable of inciting microbiallergic conjunctivitis. There is no clinical data to suggest that allergic reactions develop in the conjunctiva to viruses, although the corneal opacities of epidemic keratoconjunctivitis appear immunological in character, as do some of the corneal manifestations of herpes simplex.

Bacteria

There is little evidence that bacteria other than *Staphylococcus* play an important role in the production of allergic conjunctivitis. Apparently a combination of two factors operates in the pathogenesis of this condition: 1) chronicity, with the opportunity for repeated reinfection, and 2) antigenic exotoxins or other sensitizing substances. Most bacteria that produce potent, but not necessarily allergic, exotoxins, such as the diphtheria and tetanus bacilli, cause acute processes. Only the *Staphylococcus* appears to fill both requirements in this respect. It must be emphasized that microbiallergic conjunctivitis may occur without the presence of, or previous exposure to, what we consider pathogenic organisms. Even nonpathogenic bacteria can bring about an allergic state in certain individuals. This fact would explain the occurrence of microbiallergic conjunctivitis where only so-called nontoxin-producing *Staphylococcus epidermidis* is found.

Studies of bacteriophage typing of *Staphylococcus* by Locatcher-Khorazo and Gutierrez[2] may offer, by inference, additional confirmation of the role of bacterial allergy in staphylococcal infections. Although these authors isolated many phage types from normal eyes, it was rare to find more than one strain in the eyes of any single individual, and the same phage type was present in the nose as well. Staphylococcal ocular infections, including unilateral postoperative infections, were caused by the same type that was present in the normal eye of the same

individual. In eight postoperative infections the same phage type found before operation was found to be responsible. Repeated ocular cultures showed that the same phage type of *Staphylococcus* persisted for months, even after antibiotic therapy.

Although others have reported microbiallergic conjunctivitis due to streptococcal and gonococcal products, we have not encountered such instances.

In a detailed study of 60 incidences of all forms of conjunctival allergy (other than those due to contact allergy) investigated at the Fondation Rothschild in Paris, Morault[3] found that seven cases were due to bacterial allergy. According to her, the responsible organisms, which in some instances were multiple, were *Pneumococcus* in five cases, *S. hemolyticus* in five, *S. aureus* in three, *S. viridans* in one, colibacillus in one, and *Pseudomonas aeruginosa* in one.

Fungi

Allergic conjunctivitis due to mold spores is not uncommon. Essentially an inhalant form of allergy, like pollen allergy, the allergic reactions these fungi arouse have many of the characteristics of the immediate atopic response. *Alternaria* and *Cladosporium*, as well as yeasts, have been found to be responsible.

Other types of fungi of more pathogenic character cause allergy only after a primary infective focus has been established. Here the mechanism is of the delayed tuberculin type. The main members of this group are the dermatophytes, such as *Trichophyton* and *Candida albicans* (Monilia), which cause skin diseases. Thus, after a demonstrably infected primary dermatitis has occurred, "id" reactions may appear elsewhere. These id lesions reveal no fungi and disappear spontaneously when the original lesion is successfully treated. In the eye, such allergic reactions occur mainly as eczematous lesions affecting the eyelids; only rarely is the conjunctiva involved.

Helminths

Conjunctival allergy to intestinal parasites has been produced experimentally. Laboratory workers in this field, especially those dissecting the parasites, may contract allergic conjunctivitis from finger-to-eye contact. Reactions similar to hay fever, with conjunctivitis and asthma, also occur. Slaughterhouse workers have similar symptoms, which disappear when such exposure no longer occurs. At least two instances of recurrent allergic conjunctivitis related to *Oxyuris* infestation have been recorded.

CONTACT DERMATOCONJUNCTIVITIS

Contact allergy of the eyelids and conjunctiva constitutes by far the most common form of allergic reaction encountered in ophthalmic practice. It is generally caused by the local use of drugs; it also can be caused by cosmetics, articles of clothing, jewelry, animal or vegetable products, plastics, or chemicals used in industry. In those instances where the conjunctiva is the focal point of contact, as in the use of ophthalmic drugs, the allergic reaction usually begins as a conjunctivitis and soon involves the adjacent skin of the eyelids in a typical eczematous dermatitis. The term "contact dermatoconjunctivitis" has been applied to such a clinical picture. Where the eyelid skin is the site of the primary contact, conjunctival allergy plays little or no role in the manifestations, and an allergic eczematous dermatitis occurs without conjunctivitis. This form of reaction is usually the result of exposure to cosmetics, apparel, jewelry, metals, plants, or chemicals and is the most frequent cause of acute ocular eczema. While the allergic mechanism is basically the same, only contact dermatoconjunctivitis is discussed at this point; allergic eczematous dermatitis of the eyelids is discussed in Chapter 5.

In contact allergy of the conjunctiva, the responsible agent almost always is an ophthalmic drug. Since the conjunctiva is usually the focal point of contact, the allergic reaction generally begins as a conjunctivitis but soon involves the adjacent skin and becomes a typical contact dermatoconjunctivitis. The major diagnostic characteristics of this type of reaction in order of appearance are: 1) severe itching

of the eyes, 2) papillary conjunctivitis,, 3) eczema of the skin of the eyelids, and 4) conjunctival eosinophilia, generally developing after prolonged exposure, thus not an immediately useful diagnostic finding. If the conjunctivitis is due to eye drops, the earliest signs of eczema may be at the canthi and on the lower lids; if ointments are the offending agents, the lid margins may be involved first.

In order to prove contact allergy, patch tests are employed. They are simple to perform and very useful, especially when the patient is on multiple ocular drops, as for treatment of glaucoma. Patch testing should not be a lost art for the ophthalmologist. A patch test consists of applying a small amount of the suspected substance to a site of normal skin of the patient, covering it with an innocuous impermeable material which is sealed to the skin with adhesive, and leaving it in situ for 1 to 3 or 4 days. Sometimes one must read the reactions for as long as 5 days after the patch is removed, since the test may only then become positive. Usually contact for 24 to 48 hours is enough. The true allergic reaction increases (as a rule) in intensity for 24 to 48 hours after the patch is removed.

A negative patch test does not necessarily rule out the test substance as a causative agent, because: 1) under the test circumstances, the actual mechanism producing the inflammation may be lacking; 2) the patient may no longer be sensitive; 3) the actual sensitizer is not applied; and 4) the patient may have only a local sensitivity, and the site of skin tested is not sensitive.

It is important that the test material not be too concentrated, since it may then act as a primary skin irritant. For testing liquids, a piece of gauze one-fourth inch square is saturated. Powders are placed on moistened gauze. For solids insoluble in water, make a saturated solution in a solvent and wet some gauze with the solution, but let the gauze dry before applying it to the skin to eliminate the action of the solvent. Follow the same procedure for ointments as for liquids.

Ophthalmic tests, especially for drug allergies, should be done rarely and then with great caution. Very weak concentrations should be used, since harmful effects may occur.

ALLERGENIC DRUGS

Many ophthalmic drugs are true sensitizers. On occasion probably every drug used in the treatment of the eyes has resulted in contact dermatoconjunctivitis in some individual (Fig. 4.3). In fact, there is probably no drug or chemical in existence which everyone can use with impunity. While nonprotein substances are in themselves not primary antigens, it is believed that they form true antigens in the body by union with host tissues. These relatively simple chemicals, known as haptens, combine with body proteins, forming conjugates that act as antigens. The hapten confers specificity on the conjugate; hence, the allergy is directed against the hapten and not against the protein. This explains why the substitution of a drug that is chemically similar to one that previously caused sensitivity in a patient is dangerous. Thus, after allergy to one sulfonamide has developed, another sulfonamide is very likely to cause sensitivity. Benzamine and other chemicals with paralinked amino groups, as compared with ortho and meta attachments, are especially likely to cause contact allergies. Unfortunately, many of the drugs we use fall into that category.

Local Anesthetics

Apparently every local anesthetic used topically is a potential sensitizer, causing contact dermatoconjunctivitis. Cocaine hydrochloride, first introduced about 100 years ago by Koller, is by far the least sensitizing of all, but it has other drawbacks. At times, patients are encountered who react allergenically to all presently available topical anesthetics so that cocaine is the only local anesthetic tolerated. Succeeding anesthetics such as phenacaine (Holocaine) and piperocaine (Metycaine) were also relatively uncommon sensitizers, but caused much stinging on instillation. They were later superseded by butacaine (Butyn), which caused many allergies; dibucaine (Nupercaine), also a potent sensitizer; dimethocaine (Larocaine), the most allergenic of

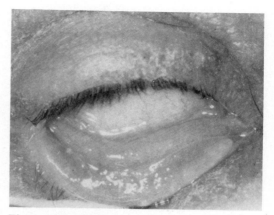

Figure 4.3 Contact dermatoconjunctivitis from eserine. (Reprinted with permission from Theodore, F.H., and Schlossman, A. Ocular Allergy. Williams & Wilkins, 1958.)

all; and tetracaine (Pontocaine), the least allergenic of this group, which is still widely used.

Proparacaine hydrochloride (Ophthaine, Ophthetic, Alcaine), an excellent anesthetic, can cause not only typical contact dermatoconjunctivitis (Fig. 4.4), but also, on occasion, may incite a hyperacute corneal reaction of the greatest severity. This is described in the chapter on allergy of the cornea (Chapter 6).

Apparently the least allergenic of currently available local anesthetics is benoxinate hydrochloride (Dorsacaine). Unfortunately, it stings more and is less effective than proparacaine, requiring several instillations for adequate anesthesia. One hyperacute corneal reaction has occurred in our experience, but contact dermatoconjunctivitis is very rare.

Antibiotics

Penicillin is notorious for its sensitizing tendencies, especially in ointment form. Streptomycin, bacitracin, the tetracyclines, chloramphenicol (Chloromycetin), erythromycin, and neomycin may all cause allergies. Neomycin is particularly important in this respect because it is used in combination with so many other antibiotics and corticosteroids. Methicillin sodium (Staphcillin) has also caused allergy.

None of the concentrated antibiotic eyedrops first introduced by Theodore in

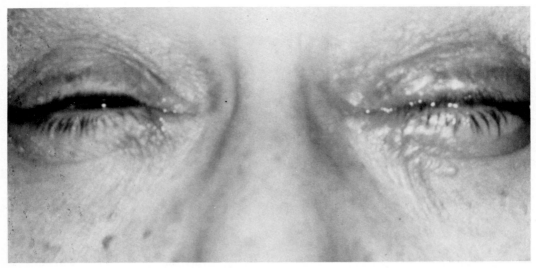

Figure 4.4 Contact dermatoconjunctivitis from proparacaine (Ophthaine). Patient had very severe corneal allergy with ulcers, as well, requiring systemic steroids.

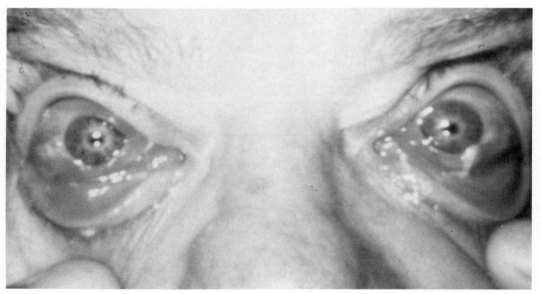

Figure 4.5 Aminoglycoside reaction in a patient treated with both neomycin and gentamicin. Reaction most probably due to latter.

1970[4] for the treatment of central corneal ulcers and postoperative endophthalmitis has caused allergy during the relatively short periods they are used, with the exception of penicillin. However, concentrated solutions of streptomycin and neomycin have caused conjunctival irritation as well as punctate epithelial keratitis that clears when the drugs are discontinued.

Similarly, subconjunctival injections of antibiotics have been surprisingly free of allergic sequelae, where drugs known to have caused allergies previously have not been used.

Special mention, however, must be made in regard to the topical use of gentamicin (Garamycin). This drug not only may cause typical contact dermatoconjunctivitis, but, more frequently, may give rise to a distinctive severe irritative reaction. Usually, the lower palpebral and adjacent bulbar conjunctiva are involved in the inflammatory process; the upper half of the eye is clear. Often the bulbar conjunctiva shows the most involvement, with localized swelling and redness lasting for weeks (Fig. 4.5). The important thing is to recognize that such a reaction may occur and to stop the drug rather than increase the frequency of its instillation in the mistaken belief that the presumed infection is worse.

Tobramycin, used topically as Tobrex, so far appears to be less allergenic and less irritating.

Antiviral Agents

Idoxuridine (IDU), available in the United States as Stoxil, Herplex and Dendrid, is a most potent sensitizer as well as a topical irritant. Usage for two or more weeks usually evokes an irritative follicular conjunctivitis. Prolonged use, or, at times, even short exposure, can result in severe contact dermatoconjunctivitis, which surprisingly is often ignored by ophthalmologists in resistant cases of herpetic keratitis due to their eagerness to heal the corneal process (Fig. 4.6). Even worse is the development of a central bacterial corneal ulcer, usually staphylococcal, but often due to other organisms. This occurs as a result of the tissue poisoning effect by this antimitotic drug as

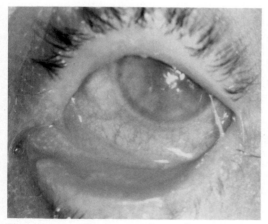

Figure 4.6 Allergy to idoxuridine showing dermatoconjunctivitis.

well as lowered immunity, whether or not corticosteroids are also being administered. Fungal ulcers may develop in a similar situation. Another toxic effect of IDU is the ground-glass corneal stippling and opacification, so common after moderately prolonged use.

Vidarabine (Vira-A, previously Ara-A) is less allergenic and irritating, but the same reactions as above may occur, although we are not aware of any instances of secondary central corneal ulcers due to infective agents. While trifluorothymidine (Viroptic) is too new to fully evaluate, so far there appears to be less allergy connected with its use. However, punctate epithelial keratitis of a temporary nature may occur, probably toxic or irritative.

Sulfonamides

All sulfonamides are prone to cause allergic reactions after prolonged topical usage.

Mydriatic and Miotic Alkaloids

Allergy to atropine is a common occurrence, resulting in a typical contact dermatoconjunctivitis with eczema, papillary conjunctivitis, and conjunctival eosinophilia. Both hyoscine and homatropine also may cause sensitivity, but the eczematous component is less evident. Atropine, however, sometimes causes follicular conjunctivitis without eosinophilia or dermatitis, due to conjunctival irritation, a different mechanism which is discussed in the next section of this chapter. An often unrecognized sensitizer is phenylephrine (Neo-Synephrine), so frequently used for office dilatation. Tropicamide (Mydriacyl) and cyclopentolate (Cyclogyl) only rarely seem to cause contact dermatoconjunctivitis.

The miotic alkaloids are rarely sensitizers. The use of pilocarpine or eserine only occasionally results in true contact dermatoconjunctivitis. Instead, the prolonged administration of these and other related synthetic miotics may produce follicular conjunctivitis, without eczema and eosinophilia, which appears to be due to drug irritation, not allergy. This will be elaborated upon later. Those very rare instances in which contact dermatoconjunctivitis as well as follicles occur, are explained by the fact that primary irritants also may be, or can become, sensitizers.

Other Common Ophthalmic Drugs

Mercurials are well-recognized sensitizers, as are drugs ranging from ethylmorphine (Dionin) hydrochloride to boric acid, including zinc salts, mild silver protein (Argyrol), and naphazoline (Privine) hydrochloride. Nitrofurazone (Furacin), quaternary ammonium compounds like benzalkonium (Zephiran) chloride, phenylephrine (Neo-Synephrine) hydrochloride, and many others may also cause allergies. Even topical corticosteroids may cause an allergy. Antihistamines used topically may cause allergies. Dermatological ointment preparations, used widely just after the introduction of these compounds, caused so many allergic reactions that they were withdrawn from the market and production abandoned.

Ophthalmic Vehicles

Preservatives used in eye solutions may be an unsuspected cause of allergy.[5, 6] This applies especially to the mercurials and to benzalkonium chloride. Ointment bases may cause allergies, usually to lanolin or petrolatum.

SYNDROME OF DRUG IRRITATION[7]

Although most cases of drug intolerance are due to drug allergy, enough instances of drug irritation occur to make it an important differential consideration. The importance of the distinction between these two types of drug reaction lies in the fact that, in drug irritations, the use of the same drug may be continued if it is prepared in a manner that prevents further irritation, while in allergies an entirely different drug must be substituted. Clinically, differentiation is generally simple.

Substances that come in contact with the skin and mucosa may be classified as 1) primary irritants or 2) cutaneous and mucosal sensitizers. Primary irritants cause inflammation by direct action at the site of contact only, if allowed to act in sufficient intensity or quantity for a long enough time. Cutaneous and mucosal sensitizers usually cause no changes on first contact, but after about 5 to 7 days the skin, or the mucous membranes, will react specifically on further contact at the original site or elsewhere. These are the sensitizers that cause contact allergy.

While some drugs are themselves primary irritants, and almost every drug may at times be irritating, conjunctivitis due to irritation usually occurs following the prolonged use of preparations that are prone to deteriorate into irritating products if not prepared in a manner that will hinder or prevent this breakdown. This process is particularly apt to occur with alkaloids. However, it should be remembered that many types of chemicals, particularly the antibiotics, are likely to cause irritative reactions. In this connection, neomycin is often an unsuspected offender, since it is used so often in combination with other antibiotics and steroids.

The clinical picture of conjunctivitis due to drug irritation is that of a nonspecific watery inflammation of the conjunctiva in which, in contrast to contact dermatoconjunctivitis, there is neither dermatitis of the eyelids nor conjunctival eosinophilia. In cases of chronic drug irritation, especially with the use of the alkaloids, follicular conjunctivitis may be the outstanding feature. The conjunctival involvement is less diffuse and less uniform than in allergy; often the area of most irritation, the lower lid and the adjacent bulbar conjunctiva, bears the brunt of the involvement. Results of skin-patch tests with these low-grade irritants are negative. In practice, it is important to know that such drugs as atropine usually cause allergies but that, on occasion, irritation may occur due to the formation of irritants like tropic acid and tropine.

The miotic alkaloids and the synthetic miotics cause irritations much more frequently than they cause allergies. However, occasional allergies are encountered, especially to aromatic compounds like pilocarpine; eserine (physostigmine); neostigmine (Prostigmin); and demecarium bromide (Humorsol), a quaternary ammonium compound containing two neostigmine molecules. Allergic reactions from diisopropylfluorophosphate or DFP (Floropryl) seem to be even more rare. The one allergic reaction to DFP we have seen proved to be due to the peanut oil vehicle. However, allergies must be expected from all miotic drugs if their use is sufficiently widespread.

The basis for the irritative, often follicular conjunctivitis, often encountered following prolonged use of miotics, appears to stem from their breakdown products, which are, of course, related to their chemical composition. All the aromatic miotics contain methyl ammonium radicals. Pilocarpine degrades to acetic acid, propionic acid, ammonia, and methylamine. Eserine forms rubeserine and methylamine through a rapid deterioration. Neostigmine appears to be more stable but irritation occurs due to the formation of dimethylamine. Demecarium bromide (Humorsol), a related drug (as noted previously), would appear to cause irritation by the same mechanism. Furtrethonium iodide (Furmethide) is another methyl ammonium agent with extremely marked irritating properties, because of which the drug is no longer available.

Two aliphatic compounds, methacholine (Mecholyl) and carbachol (choline carbamate), also contain methyl ammonium radicals that apparently break dowen to methylamine or dimethylamine. There are two other aliphatic compounds that do not contain methyl ammonium radicals—DFP and echothiophate iodide (Phospholine Iodide). Follicular reactions from DFP are not rare (Fig. 4.7). The drug degrades to hydrofluoric acid and elemental fluorine. A phosphorus derivative of choline, echothiophate iodide, appears to decompose by hydrolysis to thiocholine and diethyl ester of phosphoric acid and causes irritation, possibly on this basis.

At present, we are not aware of any instances of contact dermatoconjunctivitis from timolol maleate (Timoptic), possibly because it is new to general ophthalmic use. Topical reactions noted include irritation, possible conjunctival and corneal dryness, and superficial corneal staining in an irregular pattern.

While allergic reactions to epinephrine products used in glaucoma do occur, follicular irritative reactions appear to be more common. This drug also contains a methylamine radical. Another particularly interesting phenomenon is the deposition of clumps of melanin pigment in the interior fornix after the use of epinephrine solutions, a condition caused by the "dopa" reaction (Fig. 4.8). These compounds also pigment soft contact lenses. It may be important in some patients to use a bandage lens and an epinephrine compound. Dipivalyl epinephrine has been shown to be an L-epinephrine compound, which does not discolor a soft contact lens.[8]

In contrast, we have encountered a number of allergic reactions to phenyl-

Figure 4.7 Drug irritation due to diisopropylfluorophosphate (DFP). Note numerous follicles and absence of dermatitis. (Reprinted with permission from Theodore, F.H., and Schlossman, A. Ocular Allergy. Williams & Wilkins, 1958.)

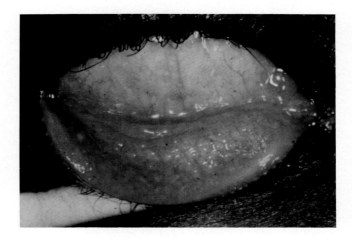

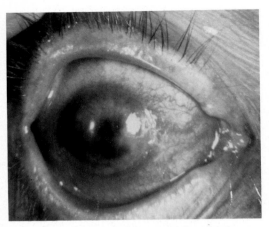

Figure 4.8 Melanin deposition in both conjunctiva and cornea in patient receiving epinephrine for longstanding glaucoma with secondary keratopathy.

ephrine (Neo-Synephrine), another methyl ammonium compound, but no characteristic irritative follicular conjunctivitis. The absence of such irritation may stem from the fact that the drug is more stable and is used less frequently in the individual patient in such high concentrations.

Drug irritation has become less of a general problem since the advent of commercially prepared ophthalmic drugs. Previously, individually compounded (drugstore) prescriptions were the source of many cases of drug irritation.

VERNAL CONJUNCTIVITIS

Vernal conjunctivitis is a recurrent, bilateral, interstitial inflammation of the conjunctiva occurring in warm weather. Although the exact cause of this disease is unknown, it is included among allergies of the eye because the condition has so many allergic features. Its possible relationship to what is called "atopic dermatitis" has long been recognized. The not infrequent occurrence of vernal conjunctivitis in patients with clear-cut evidence of atopic conjunctivitis is a definite fact. Thus the two conditions may well be expressions of one basic disease, although the conjunctivitis generally associated with atopic dermatitis has a different appearance. The effect of physical phenom-

ena such as heat and light on the precipitation of the symptoms of vernal conjunctivitis is so clear-cut that it is possible that physical allergy may be operative, with vernal conjunctivitis being an ocular reaction to the warm season in predisposed atopic individuals whose constitutions have been conditioned by a number of endocrine, metabolic, sex, and genetic factors.

Clinical Aspects

Vernal conjunctivitis is a disease of warm climates. In the Mediterranean area an incidence of up to 2% of all patients examined in eye clinics has been reported; in New York City the probable figure is less than one-tenth of 1%. In children, the condition affects boys more than three times more often than girls. After puberty the incidence is about equal in both sexes. It is a childhood disease, usually occurring from age 4 to 20.

In most patients there is a familial incidence with an allergic background more than half the time. In addition, more than 50% of all patients with vernal conjunctivitis suffer from other types of allergic diseases of an atopic nature, such as hay fever, asthma, atopic dermatitis, and allergies to foods, dust, and molds.

Blacks have been incorrectly reported in the past to be less susceptible to vernal conjunctivitis, and it was believed that when it did occur, only the limbic manifestations were noted. This is not so. Some of the most severe cases we have encountered involving extreme palpebral conjunctival manifestations and, even worse, corneal ulcerations and placques with visual impairment, are found in blacks. This is confirmed by observations among blacks in South Africa where severe permanent visual loss from this disease has been seen.

Symptoms

The outstanding symptom of the disease is extreme itching. Photophobia is also a frequent complaint.

Objective Findings

Vernal conjunctivitis is bilateral and occurs in two main forms: 1) palpebral, and 2) limbal. In a significant percentage of patients a mixed type occurs in which both the conjunctiva and the corneal limbus show changes (Fig. 4.9). The palpebral form of vernal conjunctivitis is almost always limited to the tarsal conjunctiva of the upper lid, where large cobblestone vegetations appear in longstanding cases. When the conjunctiva of the lower lid is involved, extreme severity of the condition is indicated.

The disease is essentially proliferative, characterized by a marked and continuously increasing formation of hyalinized

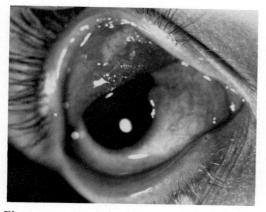

Figure 4.9 Vernal conjunctivitis: mixed type, showing palpebral and limbal involvement with thin pseudomembrane. (Courtesy of Clay-Adams Co.)

connective tissue. This opaque tissue imparts a milky, bluish appearance to the conjunctiva by obscuring the capillaries, which normally give it a pink color. In other forms of allergic conjunctivitis, regardless of how many years duration, the capillary markings are never obliterated. Sometimes patients with subjectively very severe vernal conjunctivitis may have only slight conjunctival thickening and the presence of microscopic papillae containing central blood vessels ("bloodpoints"). Usually, however, the proliferation progresses to the formation of the classical excrescences: hard, flat, large, polygonal papillae of varying size, with a predilection for the tarsus of the upper lid. In some countries, vernal conjunctivitis, because of this predominant upper lid involvement, may be confused with trachoma. When there is doubt, epithelial scrapings revealing conjunctival eosinophilia are helpful; however, the two conditions may coexist. Follicular conjunctivitis, despite its lower lid predilection, true follicular character, and preauricular adenopathy, is sometimes confused with vernal conjunctivitis.

The discharge that occurs in vernal conjunctivitis is of great diagnostic value. The tenacious, thick, "chewing-gum" pseudomembrane, which may be peeled off the conjunctiva without bleeding, is characteristic. Even if a membrane is not

Figure 4.10 Vernal conjunctivitis in patient with atopic dermatitis. Note upper palpebral vegetations.

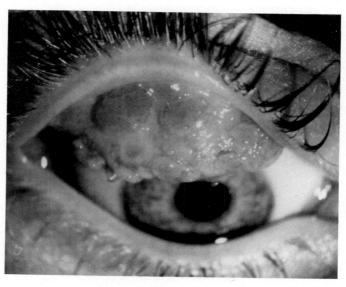

present, exposure of the everted lid, massage, or the heat of a camera light or slit lamp will result in its formation. The extremely alkaline secretion is notable for the masses of eosinophils or eosinophilic granules it contains.

The limbic proliferations of the bulbar type of vernal conjunctivitis may occur without any palpebral lesions. They appear as yellowish-gray gelatinous elevations in the palpebral fissure zone. Trantas' dots are white points which sometimes cap the excrescences and are pathognomonic of vernal conjunctivitis (Fig. 4.10). They are composed of eosinophils. As differentiated from phlyctenules, vernal lesions do not stain with fluorescein. Furthermore, there is, in general, less inflammatory reaction than in phlyctenular keratoconjunctivitis. Conjunctival eosinophilia is a valuable differential factor in determining the diagnosis.

Corneal Lesions

The most frequent and characteristic corneal lesion of vernal catarrh is a superficial epithelial keratitis, which requires biomicroscopy for its recognition and which is usually located in the upper half of the cornea. The cornea looks white, as if flour had been blown over it, and stains in a punctate fashion. These lesions clear rapidly as the condition improves (especially with the use of corticosteroids, where they may disappear in 24 to 48 hours), thus offering an excellent index of the efficacy of treatment. Other types of corneal involvement occur much less commonly; some result from direct extension of the limbal process; others are deeper and central, leaving serious opacities; still others resemble dystrophies, such as pseudogerontoxon. Keratoconus may occur in patients with vernal conjunctivitis.

Central corneal ulcerations, entirely noninfectious, may occur in vernal conjunctivitis. They generally respond to corticosteroids, especially systemic. Extensive ulcerations of a plaque-like nature with the deposition of calcific material may be encountered (as mentioned above) in blacks. These do not disappear with steroids, but persist indefinitely and eventually heal over and scar when the vernal abates with puberty (Fig. 4.11).

Diagnosis

The typical clinical picture of vernal conjunctivitis is so classical, and the history of exacerbations during the warm season so typical, that diagnosis in the United States is rarely a problem. Moreover, as noted above, the massive conjunctival eosinophilia found on epithelial scrapings is rarely if ever found in other

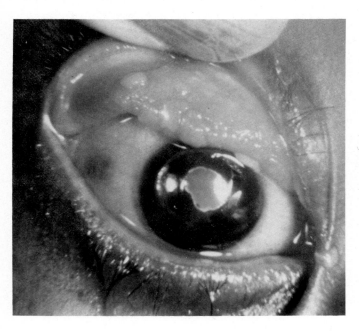

Figure 4.11 Vernal conjunctivitis with the typical palpebral vegetations and the rare plaque-like corneal ulceration with deposition of calcific material.

allergies, and certainly not in trachoma. However, the two entities may coexist. Giant papillary conjunctivitis (GPC) may resemble mild vernal, and there is sometimes a slightly eosinophilic secretion. However, the pictures are easily distinguishable, the age incidence is so different, and the history of contact lens wear is so obvious, that there can hardly be a problem except where the vernal patient uses contact lenses.

Course

Vernal conjunctivitis is almost always a childhood disease, occurring mostly from age 4 to 20. Despite the severity of the findings, and symptoms that may disable a child even in the coldest winter weather so much that he or she cannot attend school, eventually vernal conjunctivitis generally clears so completely that no indications can be perceived on ocular examination. Exceptions to this, in regard to the cornea, as noted above, are rare in the United States.

When vernal conjunctivitis occurs in adult life, the sex incidence is equal, and the condition is not self-limiting. It may go on indefinitely, as in atopic dermatitis.

Treatment

Removal of the patient to a cool environment is usually impractical and often not really effectual, unless one goes to the Southern hemisphere during the Northern summer.

The only really effective treatment of vernal is the use of corticosteroids—a tremendous advance and benefit to such patients. Where topical therapy is not effective, small doses of systemic steroids often break the cycle of symptoms. The drawback to this regime, of course, is that the risks of prolonged steroid therapy must be explained to the parents and agreed to in writing.

Treatment dosages must be judged by the parents in relation to the severity of the child's symptoms. Most importantly, regular check-ups by the ophthalmologist are mandatory.

Other treatments include: cold compresses; 1 to 2% solution of monohydrated sodium carbonate and other alkaline solutions which may dissolve or loosen mu-

cin; acetylcysteine (Mucomyst), also mucolytic, which has proved disappointing; and vasoconstrictors. Antihistamines either locally or systemically have proved ineffectual. Cromolyn sodium (Intal) is said to be of value as a substitute for steroids, once the patient is moderately well-controlled and does not need too much help.[9] Unfortunately, neither this medicament nor Mucomyst are available in the United States as commercial ophthalmic products. Any of the new modulators of cyclic AMP may eventually be of value by helping to prevent degranulation of the mast cell population.

Radiotherapy, an effective modality, was used rather extensively before the days of steroids for severe palpebral vernal but has now essentially been abandoned. Surgical removal of large vegetations has been helpful, especially where corneal complications are severe and, in addition, it facilitates elimination of the discharge. Unfortunately, the vegetations soon grow back. Simple scissors excision has proved better than cauterizing agents or cryotherapy.

CONJUNCTIVITIS ASSOCIATED WITH ATOPIC DERMATITIS

Chronic conjunctival thickening of a pale papillary appearance, with mucopurulent secretion and itching, is not uncommon in atopic dermatitis, especially when the eyelids are inflamed. Conjunctival eosinophilia is present, and S. aureus is usually grown in cultures of such eyes. Symptoms may become very severe and are best relieved by topical steroids. However, serious sequelae to this type of therapy, such as glaucoma, herpetic keratitis of great severity, and cataracts, have all been encountered by us. Cataracts, of course, were known to complicate atopic dermatitis long before the advent of steroids. The incidence of retinal detachment after cataract surgery in such patients was, and apparently still is, much higher than in other individuals.

GIANT PAPILLARY CONJUNCTIVITIS

Hard and soft contact lenses and the solutions used in their care may result in irritation and possibly allergic reactions which diminish or destroy lens wear tolerance. Giant papillary conjunctivitis (GPC), so-named and well-studied by Allansmith and her co-workers,[10] is a syndrome seen primarily in soft lens wearers that may develop relatively soon after onset of use, but on the average after 10 months. Initially, there is increased mucus and itching, followed by a satiny appearance of the upper tarsal conjunctiva, then occurrence of papillae, at first small, but eventually very large (greater than 1 mm in diameter), noted especially in the upper two-thirds of the tarsal conjunctiva (Fig. 4.12). Vision may become blurred. The onset of GPC in hard contact lens wearers appears to be a matter of many years with variable severity and much less frequency.

The papillae may resemble those of vernal conjunctivitis to some degree. Pathological studies show infiltration of the epithelium with mast cells, eosinophils, basophils and polymorphonuclear leukocytes, as well as occasional lymphocytes. In the stroma there were many lymphocytes and plasma cells, as well as eosinophils and basophils. Cytological epithelial scrapings may show eosinophils, though few in number. Deposits on the lens due to protein build-up were always noted and are hypothesized to be the antigenic incitants of this possible immunological process. Thorough cleansing of lenses, the use of new lenses (possibly of different composition), or discontinuance of lens wear entirely may be necessary to clear up the condition. Topical steroids may be used when the lenses have been discontinued. Cromolyn sodium may be of value as eye drops when lens wear is begun again.

Stenson[11] suggests that GPC may be partially mechanical in origin, occurring especially with high-riding, loose, large lenses. She states that these patients may do better with smaller, thinner, better centered lenses and meticulous edge cleaning. A mechanical origin is also suggested by the finding of GPC, unrelated to contact lens wear in patients with penetrating keratoplasties in which interrupted nylon sutures were used.[12] This has also occurred following cataract extraction due to unremoved nylon sutures. Removal of exposed sutures resolves the condition. GPC associated with the use of prostheses after enucleation has also been described.[13]

OCULAR CICATRICIAL PEMPHIGOID

The striking feature of cicatricial pemphigoid is recurrent blisters or bullae of the mucous membranes and skin with a tendency for scar formation.[14] Ocular involvement is characterized by progressive shrinkage of the conjunctiva, entropion, trichiasis, xerosis and finally reduced vision from corneal opacification.[15, 16] Cicatricial pemphigoid is essentially a disease of late life with the average age of onset being 58 years.[17] In a series of 78 patients with this disease, it was found that the ages at initial examination ranged from

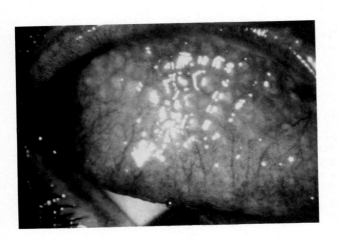

Figure 4.12 Giant papillary conjunctivitis from contact lens wear. (Stenson, S. Atlas of Conjunctival Cytology, 1979—Courtesy of Allergan Pharmaceuticals, Inc.)

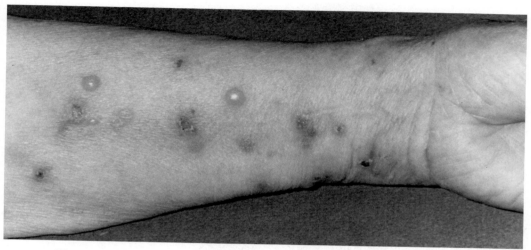

Figure 4.13 Intact and ruptured blisters of forearm in patient with OCP.

43 to 86 with a mean of 68.7 years, and that the disease affected more women than men with a ratio of 1.6 to 1.[18] Ocular cicatricial pemphigoid (OCP) is a relatively rare disease with most estimates suggesting an incidence of 1 in 20,000 to 1 in 46,000 ophthalmic cases.[15, 16] It has neither a geographic nor a racial predilection.[14]

CUTANEOUS INVOLVEMENT

The skin is involved less frequently than the mucous membranes. In an analysis of 261 patients belonging to four different series, it was found that cutaneous lesions were present in 24% of the cases.[19] Two types of skin lesions are found in this disease: 1) a recurrent, vesiculobullous, nonscarring eruption that may involve the inguinal area and the extremities and occasionally becomes generalized (Fig. 4.13), and 2) localized, erythematous plaques with vesicles and bullae that appear on the scalp and face near the affected mucous membranes and heal with smooth atrophic scars.[20]

MUCOUS MEMBRANE INVOLVEMENT

Mucous membrane involvement includes the conjunctiva, nose, oral cavity, pharynx, larynx, esophagus, anus, and vagina. An analysis of four different series containing 261 cases indicated that oral lesions were found in 91% and conjunctival lesions in 66% of patients.[19] Two

types of oral lesions are found in this disease: desquamative gingivitis and a vesiculobullous eruption.[20] The gingivitis is diffuse or patchy, heals slowly, and may persist for years without significant change. Vesicles and bullae of the oral mucosa appear rapidly and are intact for 2 to 3 days. The rupture and coalescence of these lesions may result in large areas of epithelial denudation. Rupture of submucosal blisters leaves erosions of the mucous membranes, which often heal with scarring. Scarring of the mucous membranes may lead to esophageal, urethral, vaginal, and anal strictures.

OCULAR INVOLVEMENT

The disease may appear in both eyes simultaneously or start in one and affect the other after an interval of less than 2 years.[15] Both eyes are eventually involved.

The first symptoms are those of chronic conjunctivitis with irritation, burning, and tearing. The chronic conjunctivitis may be aggravated by secondary bacterial infections, resulting in a mucopurulent discharge. Corneal involvement leads to foreign body sensation, photophobia, and finally reduced vision. An acute onset manifesting bilateral upper lid pseudomembranes and oral lesions may occur.

The essential and destructive process in OCP is fibrosis beneath the conjunctival epithelium.[15, 21, 22] As the formation of fibrous tissue progresses, symblepharon are formed, passing from the palpebral to the bulbar conjunctiva with the inferior fornix involved first. Symblepharon are best demonstrated early in the disease by drawing the lower lid down and having the patient look up, giving rise to vertical folds between the palpebral and bulbar conjunctiva (Fig. 4.14). The conjunctival shrinkage increases in extent until a condition of ankyloblepharon eventually results, with the entire conjunctival sac being obliterated (Fig. 4.15).

OCP is associated with a diminished and unstable tear film.[23] As part of the progressive submucosal shrinkage, fibrous occlusion of the ducts of the lacrimal and accessory lacrimal glands develops, leading to decreased aqueous tear secretion. Conjunctival goblet cells contribute to the mucous component of the precorneal tear film, and the destruction of these cells in OCP may result in mucin deficiency and an unstable tear film on this basis.[24, 25] Conjunctival scarring and symblepharon cause entropion with trichiasis and lagophthalmos with abnormal blinking and exposure. Because of the decreased aqueous tear secretion and decreased mucous production and lid prob-

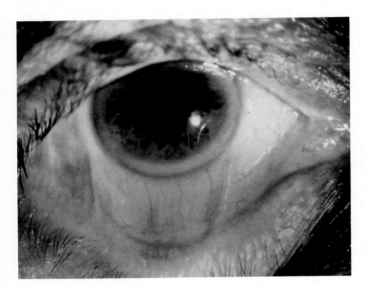

Figure 4.14 OCP: symblepharon of inferior fornix demonstrated by drawing lower lid down and having patient look up.

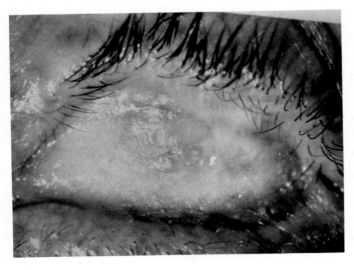

Figure 4.15 Obliteration of conjunctival fornices and keratinized ocular surface in end stage of OCP.

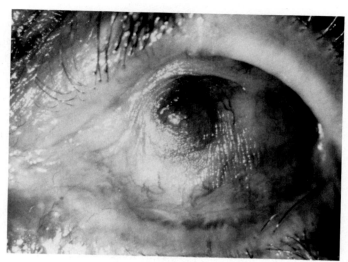

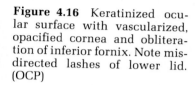

Figure 4.16 Keratinized ocular surface with vascularized, opacified cornea and obliteration of inferior fornix. Note misdirected lashes of lower lid. (OCP)

lems, the integrity of the tear film is disturbed resulting in a dry eye, with breakdown and eventual keratinization of the corneal and conjunctival epithelium (Fig. 4.16).

Decreased vision occurs as a result of corneal involvement. Primary corneal involvement with the formation of bullae of the corneal epithelium has been described.[21, 22] Erosions are believed to result from rupture of these bullae. Corneal erosions most commonly result from entropion with trichiasis, lagophthalmos with abnormal blinking and exposure, and the diminished and unstable tear film. The erosions may be complicated by secondary bacterial infiltrates and ulcers. Corneal neovascularization develops in the form of pannus and pseudopterygia. Corneal opacification results (Fig. 4.16).

Smears of the conjunctiva in OCP reveal neutrophils, keratinized squamous cells, and eosinophils.[26, 27]

In a study of the bacterial flora of patients with OCP, it was found that potential pathogens were recovered from the lids and/or conjunctiva in 49% of controls and 81% of patients with OCP.[18] On the other hand, potential pathogens were not recovered from the lids and conjunctiva of 51% of controls as opposed to 19% of patients with OCP. Mannitol positive staphylococci were the potential pathogens that were most prevalent on the lids

and conjunctiva of both controls and patients with OCP.

HISTOPATHOLOGY

Blisters or bullae are found in a subepithelial location without acantholysis.[7] Blisters of the conjunctiva probably rupture readily in this location and are only rarely observed.[21, 22] The conjunctiva shows a metaplasia of the normal columnar epithelium into squamous epithelium with parakeratinization and keratinization.[28] Mucus-producing goblet cells are scarce or absent.[25, 28] The early stages of conjunctival disease show granulation tissue beneath the conjunctival epithelium, with an infiltration predominantly of lymphocytes, plasma cells, occasional eosinophils, and relatively few polymorphonuclear leukocytes.[27, 28] Later, pronounced fibrosis takes place in the conjunctival stroma and is responsible for the conjunctival shrinkage which characterizes this disease.[21, 22]

Conjunctival biopsies in patients with acute manifestations of OCP show numerous polymorphonuclear leukocytes within and beneath the conjunctival epithelium, in addition to the chronic inflammatory cells typically found in this condition.[29]

Electron microscopic studies show that the separation at the margin of a blister is located within the lamina lucida between the plasma membrane of the basal cells and the electron-dense basal lamina.[19]

IMMUNOPATHOLOGY

In cicatrial pemphigoid, immunoglobulins and components of both the classical and alternative complement pathways are found bound to the basement membrane zone of skin and oral mucosa.[30, 31] Occasionally, circulating antibodies to the basement membrane zone can be demonstrated.

Immunoglobulins are also found bound to the basement membrane of the conjunctiva. The frequency with which conjunctival samples from patients with OCP demonstrate immunoglobulins bound to the basement membrane varies from 20 to 67%.[32-35] And so, the absence of basement membrane staining does not negate the diagnosis, but its presence would tend to confirm the clinical impression. The third component of complement has also been demonstrated bound to the conjunctival basement membrane.[34, 35] The deposition of immunoglobulins on the conjunctival basement membrane is not diagnostic of OCP but may also be found in patients with Mooren's ulcer and staphylococcal keratitis.[34] However, a more linear deposition of immunoglobulins is found with OCP while a more granular deposition is found in the other conditions.

Immunoglobulins are also found bound to the conjunctival epithelium of patients with OCP.[34, 35] Circulating antibodies which bind to the conjunctival and corneal epithelium but not to the conjunctival basement membrane have also been demonstrated.[34, 35]

The role of tissue-fixed immunoglobulins and complement in the pathogenesis of this condition is not known. Finding complement in association with immunoglobulin deposition indicates that an antibody-antigen reaction is taking place and is being increasingly recognized as important in the demonstration of an immunopathological basis for a disease. These autoimmune phenomena may be intimately involved in the pathogenesis of OCP or may simply accompany or aggravate the tissue destruction found in this disorder.

Approximately one-half of patients with OCP have elevated IgA levels.[32, 34] An association of OCP with HLA-B12 has been demonstrated, suggesting that there is an immunogenetic susceptibility to its development.[36] Patients with OCP have decreased numbers of circulating T and possibly B cells.[37]

DIFFERENTIAL DIAGNOSIS

The clinical diagnosis of OCP is essentially a diagnosis of exclusion. Radiation and severe chemical burns, particularly with alkali, may cause symblepharon and shrinkage of the conjunctiva. Adenovirus 8 and 19, primary herpes simplex keratoconjunctivitis, diphtheria and beta hemolytic streptococcus may cause a membranous conjunctivitis that results in conjunctival scarring.[33, 38] The acute, self-limited nature of these conditions contrasts with the chronic, progressive conjunctival shrinkage found with OCP.

Patients should be questioned about their medications, because symblepharon and conjunctival shrinkage have been associated with the use of systemic practolol[24] and topical epinephrine,[39] echothiophate iodide,[40] and pilocarpine.[11] Symblepharon have also been reported with Sjögren's syndrome[41] and sarcoidosis.[42] Trachoma causes conjunctival scarring but this usually begins and predominates in the superior fornix and on the upper tarsus.

Bullous pemphigoid rarely involves the conjunctiva. Although pemphigus may be associated with conjunctivitis, conjunctival shrinkage is rare. Erythema multiforme major may cause conjunctival shrinkage as a result of the acute episode, but the shrinkage is not chronically progressive as it is with OCP.

DISEASE COURSE

OCP is generally described as a chronic disease characterized by progressive shrinkage of the conjunctiva. The conjunctival shrinkage increases in extent until the entire conjunctival sac is obliterated. With absent tears, obliterated fornices, and a keratinized surface, the endstage of OCP has been reached. The chronic, progressive course of OCP may be interrupted by episodes of acute disease activity which result in rapid shrinkage of the conjunctiva.[29] In patients with OCP, surgical procedures such as lysis of symblepharon, plastic procedures on the lids and cataract extractions may entail a risk of setting off acute disease activity. The acute manifestations consist of diffuse and intense conjunctival hyperemia and edema and localized, ulcerated conjunctival mounds (Fig. 4.17). This acute inflammatory activity may be found in the absence of trichiasis and secondary bacterial infections.

In a prospective study of ocular progression in OCP, 20 patients were followed for an average of 22 months with a range of 10 to 53 months.[18] These patients were not being treated with topical corticosteroids or systemic immunosuppressives including corticosteroids. Progression in these patients was defined as increased conjunctival shrinkage. Of the 40 eyes in this series, 9 of 18 (50%) with stage 1 disease or less (25% shrinkage of the conjunctival fornices or less) showed progression. In patients with stage 2 disease (25 to 50% conjunctival shrinkage), 9 of 12 eyes (75%) showed progression. In patients with stage 3 disease (conjunctival shrinkage of approximately 75%), 7 of 9 eyes (78%) showed progression.

These results indicate that the majority of patients with OCP progress when followed for a period averaging 22 months. The results also underscore the variable course of this disease because there were patients in all stages who did not progress. Finally, these results suggest that progression is more likely to develop over a given period of time in the later stages.

TREATMENT

Artificial tears may alleviate to some extent the aqueous tear deficiency which develops. Artificial tears without preservatives are often useful if the preservatives are causing irritation or if allergies develop to them. In addition to the basic disease process, secondary bacterial infections of an acute and chronic nature complicate and aggravate this clinical condition.[39] Potential pathogens are recovered from the conjunctiva and/or lids of 81% of patients with OCP.[18] Cultures of the

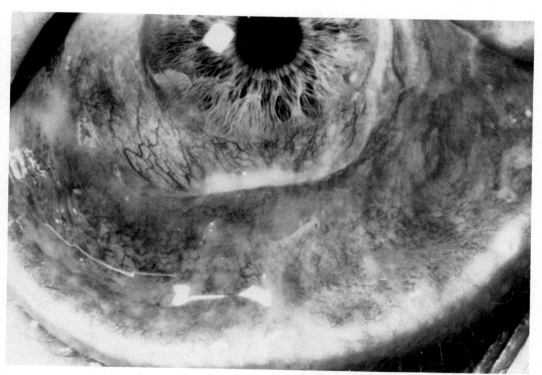

Figure 4.17 Diffuse conjunctival hyperemia and edema in OCP.

lids and conjunctiva should be performed when appropriate, and antibiotics should be prescribed on the basis of specific antibiotic sensitivity testing. The staphylococcal blepharitis which frequently accompanies this condition may be treated effectively with lid scrubs followed by an antibiotic ointment.

Entropion with trichiasis may be corrected early in the disease by oculoplastic surgical techniques but care must be taken not to shorten an already shrunken fornix. Electrolysis, cryotherapy, and hyfrecation may be used to eliminate trichiasis. When the fornices are sufficiently deep, therapeutic soft contact lenses may be used to protect the cornea from trichiasis and drying. It may be necessary to use artificial tears frequently to prevent the lens from drying. These measures do not arrest the progression of the disease, but they may keep the eye quiet and the patient comfortable in some cases.

Systemic corticosteroids are of definite value in the treatment of the acute manifestations of OCP.[29] Acute disease activity in OCP may cause rapid and alarming shrinkage of the conjunctiva. Systemic corticosteroids suppress this acute disease activity and prevent further shrinkage.

Systemic immunosuppressive treatment with prednisone and cyclophosphamide (Cytoxan) or azathioprine (Imuran) has been reported to be useful in the management of OCP.[42a] The role of diaminodiphenylsulfone (Dapsone) in treatment of OCP is not clear at present.[42b] In the final stages of OCP with ankyloblepharon and a keratinized ocular surface, a keratoprosthesis may be useful in restoring some sight to these unfortunate patients.[43]

ERYTHEMA MULTIFORME (STEVENS-JOHNSON SYNDROME)

Erythema multiforme (EM) is an acute, generally self-limited, inflammatory disorder of the skin and mucous membranes with a variable recurrent pattern. The minor form of EM primarily involves the skin. The major form is characterized by mucosal as well as cutaneous lesions, toxemia with fever and prostration, and ocular involvement. This latter variant is also known as the Stevens-Johnson syndrome.

In some studies, the diagnostic criteria for EM major do not necessarily require ocular involvement and include: 1) skin lesions; 2) erosive involvement of two or more mucous membranes; and 3) systemic toxicity, usually including malaise, fever, and prostration.[44] In the minor variant of the disease, the process may last 2 or 3 weeks, compared to 6 weeks for the major form. This disease may be seen at almost any age but peaks in the second and third decades and occurs only rarely in infancy and old age.[45] There is no racial or geographic predilection.

PRECIPITATING FACTORS

EM is considered to be a skin and mucous membrane reaction to a variety of precipitating factors. It has been related to various biological agents including viruses, bacteria, fungi, and *Mycoplasma pneumoniae*. The relationship of EM to infections with *M. pneumoniae* and herpes simplex has been the most thoroughly documented.[45] EM has been associated with primary atypical pneumonia with the demonstration of elevated titers of complement-fixing antibodies to *M. pneumoniae*. *M. pneumoniae* has even been isolated from the blister fluid of patients with EM, who also showed rising titers of complement-fixing antibodies to this agent.

Fifteen percent of patients with recurrent EM are said to experience preceding episodes of herpes simplex infections.[46] In a patient with a 7-year history of recurrent episodes of EM preceded by herpes simplex infections, intradermal skin tests with a formaldehyde-inactivated herpes simplex preparation produced bullae that were clinically and histologically interpreted as EM.[46] Not only was a local reaction triggered after the skin test, but 48 hours later a widespread vesiculobullous eruption appeared.

In one study, a history of recurrent bacterial infections that often required drainage was recorded in 20% of cases of EM major.[44] Interestingly, the classical target or iris lesions were reproduced grossly as well as microscopically in a patient with EM by the intradermal injection of a variety of heat-killed, gram-negative bacteria, as well as their common endotoxin.[47]

EM may be associated with drugs such as sulfonamides, penicillin, barbiturates, salicylates, mercurials, arsenic, phenylbutazone, and diphenylhydantoin.[44-46] Although drugs are widely accepted as etiological factors in EM, the prodromal symptoms of EM closely mimic upper respiratory tract infections that are commonly treated with antibiotics or other drugs. As a result, it is difficult to determine if the antibiotic caused EM or if the prodromal symptoms would have developed into the full-blown syndrome even in the absence of the drug. Recurrences of EM on rechallenge with sulfonamides or other suspected drugs have been documented.[48] EM has been reported following the use of topical ophthalmic scopolamine, tropicamide, and sulfonamides.[49]

Thirty-one percent of patients have been reported to have a past history of atopic disorders or laboratory evidence of autoimmune disease such as antinuclear antibodies or rheumatoid factor.[44] EM has also been related to radiation therapy, malignancy, and collagen-vascular diseases.[50]

CLINICAL MANIFESTATIONS

The prodromal symptoms of EM include malaise, fever, symptoms of upper respiratory tract infection, prostration, and headache. Mucous membrane and skin involvement follow. The cutaneous lesions are most frequently found on the extremities and, except for the more severe cases, spare the trunk. The cutaneous lesions have a predilection for the dorsal aspect of the hands and feet as well as the extensor surfaces of the forearms and legs. The skin lesions develop in crops and are symmetrically distributed. They begin as erythematous macules and papules, progress to become vesicles and bullae, and resolve leaving residual hyperpigmentation. The characteristic lesion of EM is the target lesion. This consists of a red center surrounded by a pale zone with another red ring peripheral to the pale zone. Tense bullae develop from these lesions. The skin lesions are usually symptomless but are associated occasionally with burning or itching (Fig. 4.18).

Severe mucosal involvement is found in the major form of EM. Although all mucous membranes may be involved, the mouth and eyes are most frequently and severely affected. In a study of predominant clinical features of EM major over a 10-year period, it was found that 100% of patients showed stomatitis while 63% showed conjunctivitis and 61% showed balanitis, vaginitis, or urethritis.[44] The lips may be swollen and crusted but the gingivae are usually spared. Oral lesions begin as small erythematous macules, lasting a few hours before developing into clear or hemorrhagic bullae.[45] Within 2 days a slough of the necrotic epithelium overlying the bulla is noted, resulting in an inflamed, painful hemorrhagic base with a white pseudomembrane. During the ensuing week epithelialization occurs. The process may extend to the ex-

Figure 4.18 Skin rash and respiratory distress in a patient with EM caused by administration of systemic sulfonamide.

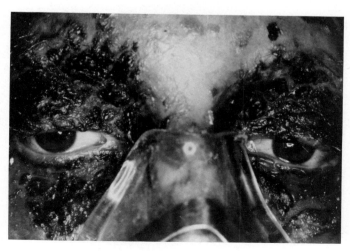

ternal nares, pharynx, larynx, trachea, bronchi, and esophagus. Except for the conjunctiva, mucosal and cutaneous lesions usually disappear without scarring.

Complications of EM include pneumonitis, septicemia, myocarditis, myositis, and acute glomerulonephritis. The reported mortality is less than 1% for EM minor and 2 to 25% for EM major.[51] Recurrences occur in about 20% of cases of both EM minor and major.[51]

OCULAR INVOLVEMENT

The acute phase of ocular disease lasts 2 to 3 weeks.[52] The lids are swollen, ulcerated, and crusted. Conjunctival vesicles have been reported.[53,54] Conjunctival involvement ranges from a mild catarrhal

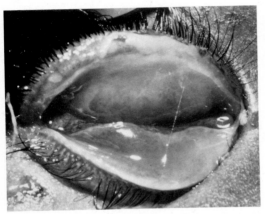

Figure 4.19 Membranes of palpebral conjunctiva in a patient with EM.

conjunctivitis which terminates without sequelae to pseudomembranous or membranous conjunctivitis. Membranes and pseudomembranes may be found on both the palpebral and bulbar conjunctiva (Fig. 4.19). Secondary bacterial infections may be responsible for the development of a purulent conjunctivitis. The conjunctival surfaces heal with scarring and symblepharon, which may even progress to ankyloblepharon. Conjunctival scarring may result in entropion with trichiasis and lagophthalmos with exposure. Obliteration of the lacrimal puncta and canaliculi by fibrosis may cause epiphora in some patients. Destruction of conjunctival goblet cells and fibrotic obstruction of the ducts from the lacrimal and accessory lacrimal glands may result in a dry eye condition similar to OCP. In severe cases, keratinization of the conjunctival and corneal epithelium may be found. The dry eye condition and entropion with trichiasis result in corneal complications that include punctate erosions, pannus, ulcers, opacification, and even perforation[52-54] (Fig. 4.20). An anterior uveitis has been described with EM.[52-54]

It has been reported that the severity of systemic disease and conjunctival involvement and not local treatment determine the severity of late ophthalmic complications.[55] Patients with pseudomembranous or membranous conjunctivitis tend to develop late ophthalmic complications.

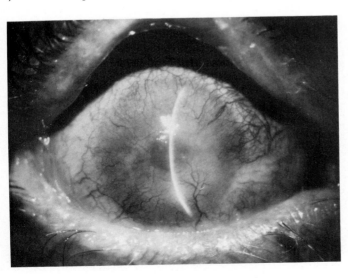

Figure 4.20 Corneal neovascularization and opacification resulting from EM.

Recurrences of EM major do not commonly involve the conjunctiva. And so EM leaves conjunctival shrinkage and symblepharon in its wake, but progressive scarring does not occur once the acute stage has subsided, unlike the chronic, progressive course of OCP. Further destruction of the eye depends upon complications resulting from the acute event, such as entropion with trichiasis and the dry eye condition with its propensity for secondary bacterial infections. These complications may result in chronically hyperemic eyes with a tendency for breakdown of the corneal epithelium that may eventuate in corneal ulcers and even perforations.

HISTOPATHOLOGY

The skin lesions of EM invariably show a mononuclear cell infiltrate in the dermis, predominantly in a perivascular location.[56] The perivascular cellular infiltrate contains mainly lymphocytes and histiocytes with occasional eosinophils and extravasated erythrocytes and rare neutrophils.[45] In addition, dermal edema and intercellular edema of the epidermis often occur with microvesiculation at the junction of the epidermis and dermis. The bullae of EM are subepithelial with adjacent lymphocytes, histiocytes, and a few neutrophils or eosinophils.[57] The basement membrane may form the roof or the floor of a bulla. Electron microscopic studies of dermal vessels have shown enlargement and vacuolization of endothelial cells as well as abnormalities of the vascular basal lamina.[45] A true necrotizing vasculitis is not found.

In a study of biopsy specimens from nonulcerated areas of the mouth in 25 patients with EM, the lamina propria showed edema, vascular dilatation, and inflammatory infiltrate, which was both perivascular and diffuse in the upper portions of the lamina propria and primarily perivascular in its deeper portion.[58] The inflammatory infiltrate was composed mainly of mononuclear cells but also contained neutrophils and/or eosinophils in almost half of the cases.

A chronic nonspecific inflammatory reaction of the conjunctiva is found with a perivascular infiltration of lymphocytes.[53]

Pseudomembranes may form from the fibrinous exudate, inflammatory cells, and necrotic epithelial cells. In some cases with severe necrotizing reactions, true membranes result from sloughing of the conjunctival epithelium and subepithelial layer.

IMMUNOPATHOLOGY

Recent studies have demonstrated circulating immune complexes in the sera of patients with EM.[50, 56, 58-60] In addition, direct immunofluorescent studies of the involved skin of patients with EM have shown deposition of C3, IgM, fibrin, and occasionally IgG in the blood vessel walls of the dermis.[50, 56, 58-60] Immunoglobulin and complement deposition is not found in blood vessel walls of the dermis in normal, unaffected skin from patients with EM, although they can be caused to deposit there by injection of histamine.[56] After histamine injection in these patients biopsies of normal skin revealed granular deposits of C3 lodged in the microvasculature of the middermis. This finding suggested that the immune complexes in EM are probably circulating and do not form locally in the tissue.

The sera of patients with EM tested by indirect immunofluorescence are negative for skin-reactive antibodies.[50] Patients with EM do not show complement deposition along or circulating antibodies to the basement membrane zone of skin.

Patients with EM major with ocular involvement have an increased prevalence of HLA-Bw 44 (a subdivision of B12).[61]

TREATMENT

There is no specific treatment presently available for this disease of unknown pathogenesis. It is of prime importance to eliminate any suspected etiological factors. Nonessential drugs should be discontinued.

EM minor requires little treatment in most cases. Wet dressings may be used to debride crusted erosions, and baths may minimize discomfort.[45] With severe and extensive cutaneous and mucosal involvement, hydration may be necessary to maintain fluid balance and analgesics may be needed to relieve pain. Local mouth care includes warm saline mouth-washes, topical anesthetics and topical corticosteroids.[45] The systemic administration of antibiotics is indicated for underlying infection. Systemic corticosteroids have been recommended for the general manifestations of EM.[45] A typical regimen consists of an initial dose of 60 to 80 mg of prednisone daily until improvement is noted, with gradual tapering over 3 to 4 weeks. The value of systemic corticosteroids has not been proven by a well-controlled, prospective study and has thus been challenged. A retrospective review of 32 children with EM major suggests that the group treated with systemic corticosteroids had a prolonged recovery with a striking incidence of medical complications compared to the group receiving only supportive care.[62]

Local treatment appears to have little influence on the severity of ophthalmic complications.[55] Early lysis of symblepharon does not appear to be effective.[23] Secondary bacterial infections of the conjunctiva should be treated by appropriate antibiotics. The dry, scarred eye resulting from EM major may require artificial tears, closure of the lacrimal puncta, destruction of aberrant lashes by electrolysis or cryotherapy, soft contact lenses to protect the cornea from drying and trichiasis, and lid scrubs followed by antibiotic ointment for the chronic blepharitis that is often found with this disease.

CONJUNCTIVAL EOSINOPHILIA AND BASOPHILIA

In laboratory diagnosis of conjunctival allergy, epithelial scrapings, preferably stained by the Giemsa method, are often of great value because they may reveal the presence of eosinophils or eosinophilic granules (sometimes in great number) as well as basophils (less frequently and fewer in number).[63] Antigen combined with IgE attached to basophils or their tissue counterparts, the mast cells, actually mediates the allergic reaction by releasing a number of inflammatory products, including histamine, other inflammatory mediators, and eosinophilic chemotactic factor of anaphylaxis (ECF-

Table 4.2
Conjunctival Eosinophilia and Basophilia

1. Vernal conjunctivitis (during remissions eosinophilia may diminish, while basophils may increase in number).
2. All types of acute and chronic allergic conjunctivitis (except bacterial allergy).
3. Conjunctivitis associated with atopic dermatitis
4. Severe chemical or vegetable irritants (lye, lime, ipecac, insect powder, indelible pencil, ricin, turpentine) may result in massive eosinophilia. This is encountered in industry or as a self-induced conjunctivitis (malingering).
5. Conjunctival parasites, myiasis, insects, hornet stings, sporotrichosis, and trypanosomiasis.
6. Ocular cicatricial pemphigoid (later stages).

Conjunctival eosinophilia does not occur in drug intolerance due to drug irritation, such as is encountered with the miotic alkaloids and the synthetic miotics. Neither does it occur in phlyctenular keratoconjunctivitis, a valuable point in the differentiation of this condition from the limbic form of vernal conjunctivitis.

A). The probable explanation for the presence of eosinophils in allergic reactions is that they modulate these released inciting agents. As far as the patient is concerned, release of these mediators from basophils and mast cells results in the sudden onset of symptoms of ocular allergy.

Eosinophils usually are not seen early in the onset of allergy, or for that matter early in OCP, but may be encountered more frequently and more abundantly in allergies of longer standing. It may be observed that in stained conjunctival scrapings, eosinophils are often not as distinctive as in blood smears and may be missed in cursory microscopic studies. The failure to find eosinophils or eosinophilic granules does not rule out allergy.

Table 4.2 lists the causes of conjunctival eosinophilia and basophilia.

REFERENCES

1. Theodore, F.H., Schlossman, A. Ocular Allergy. Williams & Wilkins, Baltimore, 1958.
2. Locatcher-Khorazo, D., Gutierrez, E. Bacteriophage typing of *Staphylococcus aureus*: A study

of normal, infected eyes and environment. Arch. Ophthalmol. 63:774–787, 1960.

3. Morault, S. Enquête allergologique et traitement par desensibilisation spécifique dans les conjunctivitis allergiques. Thése pour le doctorate en Médecine. Faculté de Médecine de Paris, July 6, 1959.

4. Theodore, F.H. Points in the Treatment of Bacterial Corneal Ulcers. Symposium on Ocular Therapy, 1970, edited by Leopold, I.H. C.V. Mosby, St. Louis, pp. 148–154, 1972.

5. Theodore, F.H., Feinstein, R.R. Practical suggestions for the preparation and maintenance of sterile ophthalmic solutions. Am. J. Ophthalmol. 35:656–659, 1952.

6. Theodore, F.H., Feinstein, R.R. Preparation and maintenance of sterile ophthalmic solutions. J. Am. Med. Assoc. 152:1631–1633, 1953.

7. Theodore, F.H. Drug sensitivities and irritations of the conjunctiva. J. Am. Med. Assoc. 151:25–30, 1953.

8. Newton, M.J., Nesburn, A.B. Lack of hydrophilic lens discoloration in patients using dipivalyl epinephrine for glaucoma. Am. J. Ophthalmol. 87:193–195, 1979.

9. Easty, D.R., Rice, N.S.C., Jones, B.R. Disodium cromoglycate in the treatment of vernal conjunctivitis. Trans. Ophthalmol. Soc. U.K. 91:491, 1971.

10. Allansmith, M.R., Korb, D.R., Greiner, J.V., Henriquez, A.S., Simon, M.A., Finnemore, V.M. Giant papillary conjunctivitis in contact lens wearers. Am. J. Ophthalmol. 83:697, 1977.

11. Stenson, S. Personal communication.

12. Sugar, A., Meyer, R.F. Giant papillary conjunctivitis after keratoplasty. Am. J. Ophthalmol. 91:239–242, 1981.

13. Srinivasan, B.D., Jakobiec, F.A., Iwamoto, T., DeVoe, A.G. Giant papillary conjunctivitis with ocular prosthesis. Arch. Ophthalmol. 97:892, 1979.

14. Rook, A., Wilkinson, D.S., Ebling, F.J.G. Textbook of Dermatology, vol. II. Blackwell, Oxford, pp. 1163–1192, 1968.

15. Duke-Elder, S. Diseases of the outer eye. Conjunctiva. In System of Ophthalmology, vol. 8, part I. C.V. Mosby, St. Louis, pp. 498–527, 1965.

16. Smith, R.C., Myers, E.A., Lamb, H.D. Ocular and oral pemphigus. Arch. Ophthalmol. 11:635, 1934.

17. Hardy, K.M., Perry, H.O., Pingree, G.C., Kirby, T.J. Benign mucous membrane pemphigoid. Arch. Dermatol. 104:467, 1971.

18. Mondino, B.J., Brown, S.I. Ocular cicatricial pemphigoid. Ophthalmology 88:95, 1981.

19. Lever, W.F. Pemphigus and pemphigoid. J. Am. Acad. Dermatol. 1:2, 1979.

20. Moschella, S.L., Pillsbury, D.M., Hurley, H.J. Dermatology, vol. I. W.B. Saunders, Philadelphia, pp. 460–476, 1975.

21. Gazala, J.R. Ocular pemphigus. Am. J. Ophthalmol. 48:355, 1959.

22. Klauder, J.V., Cowan, A. Ocular pemphigus and its relation to pemphigus of the skin and mucous membranes. Am. J. Ophthalmol. 25:643, 1942.

23. Baum, J.L. Systemic disease associated with tear deficiencies. Int. Ophthalmol. Clin. 13:157, 1973.

24. Jones, D.B. Prospects in the management of tear deficiency states. Trans. Am. Acad. Ophthalmol. Otolaryngol. 83:693, 1977.

25. Ralph, R.A. Conjunctival goblet cell density in normal subjects and in dry eye syndromes. Invest. Ophthalmol. 14:299, 1975.

26. Mondino, B.J. Bullous diseases of the skin and mucous membranes. In Clinical Ophthalmology, edited by Duane, T., vol. 4. Harper & Row, Philadelphia, Ch. 12, pp. 1–16, 1980.

27. Norn, M.S., Kristensen, E.B. Benign mucous membrane pemphigoid II. Cytology. Acta Ophthalmol. 52:282, 1974.

28. Andersen, S.R., Jensen, O.A., Kristensen, E.B., Norn, M.S. Benign mucous membrane pemphigoid III. Biopsy. Acta Ophthalmol. 52:455, 1974.

29. Mondino, B.J., Brown, S.I., Lempert, S., Jenkins, M.S. The acute manifestations of ocular cicatricial pemphigoid: Diagnosis and treatment. Ophthalmology 86:543, 1979.

30. Griffith, M.R., Fukuyama, K., Tuffanelli, D., Silverman, S. Immunofluorescent studies in mucous membrane pemphigoid. Arch. Dermatol. 109:195, 1974.

31. Rogers, R.S., Perry, H.O., Bean, S.F., Jordan, R.E. Immunopathology of cicatricial pemphigoid. Studies of complement deposition. J. Invest. Dermatol. 68:39, 1977.

32. Bean, S.F., Furey, N., West, C.E., Andrews, T., Esterly, N.B. Ocular cicatricial pemphigoid. Trans. Am. Acad. Ophthalmol. Otolaryngol. 81:806, 1976.

33. Furey, N., West, C., Andrews, T., Paul, P.D., Bean, S.F. Immunofluorescent studies of ocular cicatricial pemphigoid. Am. J. Ophthalmol. 80:825, 1975.

34. Mondino, B.J., Brown, S.I., Rabin, B.S. Autoimmune phenomena of the external eye. Ophthalmology 85:801, 1978.

35. Mondino, B.J., Ross, A.N., Rabin, B.S., Brown, S.I. Autoimmune phenomena in ocular cicatricial pemphigoid. Am. J. Ophthalmol. 83:443, 1977.

36. Mondino, B.J., Brown, S.I., Rabin, B.S. HLA antigens in ocular cicatricial pemphigoid. Arch. Ophthalmol. 97:479, 1979.

37. Mondino, B.J., Rao, H., Brown, S.I. T and B lymphocyte enumerations in ocular cicatricial pemphigoid. Am. J. Ophthalmol. 92:536–542, 1981.

38. Darougar, S., Quinlan, M.P., Gibson, J.A., Jones, B.R., McSwiggan, D.A. Epidemic keratoconjunctivitis and chronic papillary conjunctivitis in London due to Adenovirus type 19. Br. J.

Ophthalmol. 61:76, 1977.

39. Kristensen, E.B., Norn, M.S. Benign mucous membrane pemphigoid. 1. Secretion of mucus and tears. Acta Ophthalmol. 52:266, 1974.

40. Patten, J.R., Cavanagh, H.D., Allansmith, M.R. Induced ocular pseudopemphigoid. Am. J. Ophthalmol. 82:272, 1976.

41. Jones, B.R. The ocular diagnosis of benign mucous membrane pemphigoid. Proc. R. Soc. Med. 54:109, 1961.

42. Flach, A. Symblepharon is sarcoidosis. Am. J. Ophthalmol. 85:210, 1978.

42a. Foster, C.S., Wilson, L.A., Ekins, M.B. Immunosuppressive therapy for progressive ocular cicatricial pemphigoid. Ophthalmology 89:340–352, 1982.

42b. Rogers, R.S., Seehafer, J.R., Perry, H.O.: Treatment of cicatricial (benign mucous membrane) pemphigoid with dapsone. J. Am. Acad. Dermatol. 6:215–223, 1982.

43. Rao, G.N., Blatt, H.L., Aquavella, J.V. Results of keratoprosthesis. Am. J. Ophthalmol. 88:190, 1979.

44. Yetiv, J.Z., Bianchine, J.R., Owen, J.A. Etiologic factors of the Stevens-Johnson syndrome. South. Med. J. 73:599, 1980.

45. Tonnesen, M.G., Soter, N.A. Erythema multiforme. J. Am. Acad. Dermatol. 1:357, 1979.

46. Shelley, W.B. Herpes simplex virus as a cause of erythema multiforme. J. Am. Med. Assoc. 201:71, 1967.

47. Shelley, W.B. Bacterial endotoxin (lipopolysaccharide) as a cause of erythema multiforme. J. Am. Med. Assoc. 243:58, 1980.

48. Kauppinen, K. The clinical study of cutaneous reactions to drugs. Acta Derm. Venereol. (Supple) 52:5, 1972.

49. Guill, M.A., Goette, D.K., Knight, C.G., Peck, C.C., Lupton, G.P.: Erythema multiforme and urticaria. Eruptions induced by chemically related ophthalmic anticholinergic agents. Arch. Dermatol. 115:742, 1979.

50. Bushkell, L.L., Mackel, S.E., Jordon, R.E. Erythema multiforme: Direct immunofluorescence studies and detection of circulating immune complexes. J. Invest. Dermatol. 74:372, 1980.

51. Chanda, J.J. Erythema multiforme. Perspect. Ophthalmol. 3:183, 1979.

52. Dohlman, C.H., Doughman, D.J. The Stevens-Johnson syndrome. In Symposium on Cornea. Transactions of the New Orleans Academy of Ophthalmology. C.V. Mosby, St. Louis, pp. 236–252, 1972.

53. Howard, G.M. The Stevens-Johnson syndrome. Ocular prognosis and treatment. Am. J. Ophthalmol. 55:893, 1963.

54. Patz, A. Ocular involvement in erythema multiforme. Arch. Ophthalmol. 43:244, 1950.

55. Arstikaitis, M.J. Ocular aftermath of Stevens-Johnson syndrome. Arch. Ophthalmol. 90:376, 1973.

56. Wuepper, K.D., Watson, P.A., Kazmierowksi, J.A. Immune complexes in erythema multiforme and the Stevens-Johnson syndrome. J. Invest. Dermatol. 74:368, 1980.

57. Korting, G.W., Deak, R. Differential Diagnosis in Dermatology. W.B. Saunders, Philadelphia, pp. 421–422, 1976.

58. Buchner, A., Lozada, F., Silverman, S. Histopathologic spectrum of oral erythema multiforme. Oral. Surg. 49:221, 1980.

59. Hugg, J.C., Weston, W.L., Carr, R.I. Mixed cryoglobulinemia, ^{125}I C1q binding and skin immunofluorescence in erythema multiforme. J. Invest. Dermatol. 74:375, 1980.

60. Imamura, S., Uanase, K., Taniguchi, S., Ofuji, S., Mangaoil, L. Erythema multiforme: Demonstration of immune complexes in the sera and skin lesions. Br. J. Dermatol. 102:161, 1980.

61. Mondino, B.J., Brown, S.I., Biglan, A. HLA Antigens in the Stevens-Johnson syndrome with ocular involvement. Arch. Ophthalmol. 100:1453–1454, 1982.

62. Rasmussen, J.E. Erythema multiforme in children. Response to treatment with systemic corticosteroids. Br. J. Dermatol. 95:181, 1976.

63. Theodore, F.H. The significance of conjunctival eosinophilia in the diagnosis of allergic conjunctivitis. Eye, Ear, Nose Throat Monthly 30:653, 1951.

CHAPTER FIVE

The Eyelids

The eyelid is often the site of allergic reactions. In fact, such allergies occur so often that they would appear to constitute, at least statistically, the most important form of ocular allergy encountered in clinical practice. Because the eyelids represent a transitional structure consisting of conjunctiva and skin with lid margin between, allergies of both the conjunctiva and the eyelids often overlap and occur at the same time. The most important such combined allergic reaction, contact dermatoconjunctivitis, has already been described. Table 5.1 classifies all types of allergic reactions of the eyelids that are encountered.

ALLERGIC EDEMA OF THE EYELIDS

Anaphylactic and atopic allergic reactions of the eyelids basically manifest themselves as urticaria or edema of the lids. Reactions may occur in serum sickness, from insect bites, from the ingestion of all types of foods and many drugs, and sometimes, although rarely, from inhalants and contactants. Even microbial allergens, particularly fungal products, may cause urticarial reactions about the eyelids. In addition, physical agents, such as cold or sunlight, may result in such urticaria. The underlying mechanism of all the urticarias involves the localized increase in vascular permeability that occurs through the release of vasoactive mediators, mainly histamine, from mast cells or basophils to which IgE and antigen are fixed.

CONTACT ALLERGY OF THE EYELIDS

The skin of the eyelids is particularly susceptible to allergic inflammation for several special reasons. First, its fine texture and extreme thinness readily permit minor traumatization and the penetration of noxious substances of all types. Second, because of their location, the eyelids are especially exposed to physical trauma (rubbing, heat, sun, wind, and ocular secretions) and to various drugs and chemicals applied elsewhere on the head and face. Thus, although a facial cream or hair tonic is not directly applied to the eyelids, the eyelids may eventually prove to be the only site of the eczema, since even a minimal amount of the irritant, indirectly contacted by means of the fingers or from a pillowcase during sleep, is able to penetrate sufficiently to cause the reaction, in contrast to its inability to penetrate the thicker and stronger skin where it was originally applied so generously. Similarly, the skin of the eyelids often reacts to bacterial products or ocular medicaments occurring in tears which would be harmless elsewhere on the skin.

Contact allergy of the eyelids is usually due to the use of cosmetics or ophthalmic drugs.[1] Allergy to plants, however, is not uncommon. Less often, articles of apparel, jewelry, metals, plastics, other chemicals, as well as various animal and vegetable products too numerous to mention, may cause a reaction. The relative importance of the various contactants causing allergic eczematous dermatitis is difficult to evaluate. However, it appears clear that cosmetics and drugs are the two major offenders. The dermatitis, which may be either unilateral or bilateral, occurs mostly in women, probably more because they use cosmetics than because of any endocrine factor. There need be no previous history of familial or personal allergy. The diagnosis is based on a carefully taken history, a positive patch test, and a ruling out of other major causes of eyelid eczema, namely, primary ocular infection or generalized dermatoses. In addition, one must be certain that the contact dermatitis present is due to allergy rather than to primary irritation. The highlight of therapy is to eliminate the sensitizing agent; the use of any other allergenic substance may aggravate the condition seriously.

The mechanism for the production of contact allergy has been fairly well established. The site of eczematous (contact type) allergic dermatitis appears to be strictly superficial, not deeper in the skin. For this reason, in order to prove contact allergy, patch tests are necessary. Immediate wheal testing by intradermal injections is not a correct diagnostic procedure, because even the most superficial intracutaneous or scratch test carries the allergen through the epidermis into the cutis.

The etiological agent is often a simple chemical of low molecular weight that acts as a hapten by combining firmly and irreversibly with tissue protein to form a complete antigen (immunogen). The predominant response in nonatopic patients is cell-mediated (delayed) hypersensitivity by sensitized lymphocytes.

Table 5.1
Clinical Reactions of the Eyelids

I. Anaphylactic and atopic allergy (immediate)
   A. Allergic edema (urticaria, angioneurotic edema, serum sickness): drugs, animal sera, insect bites, etc.
II. Contact allergy (delayed)
   A. Contact dermatoconjunctivitis: drugs, chemicals
   B. Eczematous contact dermatitis: cosmetics, drugs, chemicals, apparel
III. Microbial allergy may play a role in:
   A. Infectious eczematoid dermatitis
      1. Bacterial: staphylococci, streptococci
      2. Fungal: trichophytosis, moniliasis
   B. Infections of the lid margin (usually staphylococcal)
      1. Blepharitis
      2. Meibomitis
      3. Hordeolum
      4. Chalazion

Ophthalmic Medicaments

Most instances of contact allergy to topical medicaments begin in the conjunctiva, as it is generally the focal point of contact of the drug. However, certain medicaments that are directly applied to the skin of the eyelids do not cause conjunctivitis (Fig. 5.1). These include antiseptics such as iodine, picric acid, mercurials, benzalkonium (Zephiran) chloride, boric acid, and witch hazel. However, most of the time ointments are the prime offenders, especially those ointments used to relieve itching or irritation of the eyelids and particularly those containing anesthetics, antihistaminics (Fig. 5.2), or even corticosteroids. Reactions may occur from the use of all types of adhesive tape (Fig. 5.3).

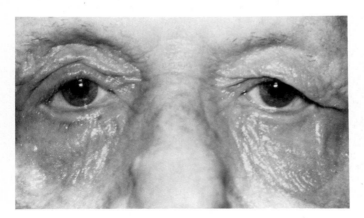

Figure 5.1 Contact dermatitis with ectropion caused by topically applied ointment containing neomycin. Patch tests showed delayed hypersensitivity to neomycin and condition resolved with discontinuation of ointment.

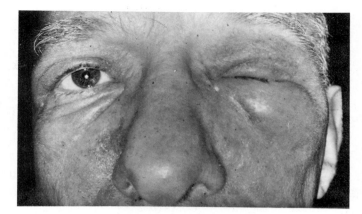

Figure 5.2 Allergy to antihistamine ointment.

Cosmetics

Cosmetics have been used widely for thousands of years despite sporadic unsuccessful attempts to outlaw the custom, such as the introduction of a bill in the British Parliament in the 18th century proposing to make the beguiling of men into matrimony by their use punishable, as for witchcraft. So much is now known about the action of cosmetics on the skin, and the exclusion of harmful ingredients is so regulated by law, that the reasons for their use far outweigh the occasional harm that occurs. Actually, if one considers how universally cosmetics are used, the incidence of allergies to them is extremely low.

Unlike drug allergy, cosmetic allergy usually begins by involvement of the upper lid, especially at the medial portion. Generally the conjunctiva is uninflamed and without eosinophilia. In the diagnosis of eyelid eczema due to cosmetics, it must be remembered that only the eyelids may react even though the allergenic substance was applied far from them. Careful history taking is essential; the use of leading questions often is important in opening avenues of thought otherwise dismissed by the patient as immaterial. Just because a cosmetic has been used previously for a long time without reaction, it should not be completely exonerated, because the manufacturer may have changed the composition or production method in some way. In diagnostic testing

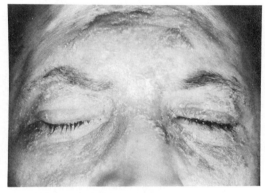

Figure 5.3 Allergy to adhesive tape. (Courtesy of Clay-Adams, Inc.)

for cosmetic sensitivity it is better to apply the cosmetic as it is ordinarily used instead of doing a patch test, because in normal use the uncovered cosmetic loses most of its substance by evaporation. Covering the cosmetic with a patch does not permit this evaporation and may give rise to false-positive reactions with cosmetics that are actually harmless when used in the ordinary manner.

Most present day allergies to cosmetics are due to the perfumes used and to impurities in manufacture, because the previously most flagrant offenders have been eliminated. Sometimes, while the cosmetic itself is innocent, contamination of the containers may cause allergies. A few important types of cosmetics which produce allergies follow.

Nail Polish and Nail Lacquer

Allergy to nail polish and nail lacquer once was extremely common but is now less frequent (Fig. 5.4). The offending ingredients are believed to be the synthetic resins, such as methacrylates, and possibly the dyes.

Face Powders

Face powders used to be sensitizers because of the orris root and the rice powder content. These ingredients are rarely used at present, having been replaced by titanium salts. Now any allergy to face powder is usually traced to perfumes and to impurities in manufacture and packaging.

Facial Creams

Facial creams such as plain cold cream and vanishing creams are not often sensitizers. In both, the major offender is either lanolin or cocoa butter and almond oil. Emulsifying agents and perfumes should also be suspected.

Lipstick

Lipstick dermatitis is usually due to the indelible dyes used.

Perfumes

The extremely complicated nature of perfumes makes such products especially liable to cause allergies. Their highly frequent use, not only alone but also to make other products more attractive, makes perfumes a common cause of contact allergy.

Hair Preparations

Hair dyes and rinses contain both sensitizers and toxic products. The most commonly used ingredient, paraphenylenediamine, may be both toxic and allergenic. Generally, allergies occur from its use, but in susceptible persons serious toxic reactions may develop. Paraphenylenediamine is also the major sensitizer in allergy to furs. Metallic dyes may cause allergies; vegetable dyes are safer. Hair tonics and lotions also contain other sensitizing agents.

Other Causes of Contact Allergy of the Eyelids

Wearing apparel, using dyed fabrics, especially if the dyes tend to "bleed" or come out of the fabric easily, can cause allergy, as can the materials used for laundering and dry cleaning. Allergy to leather is usually due to the manufacturing process. Shoe polishes and shoe dyes may cause severe allergy. Furs may cause allergic dermatitis of the eyelids because of the dyes used in their manufacture. Allergy to jewelry is not uncommon, particularly to the metals, such as nickel, cobalt, platinum, copper, chromium, aluminum, and gold used in jewelry. Spectacle frames may cause allergies, and in most reported cases of such, the frame has been of the metallic (white gold) type, with the nickel content responsible for the allergic reaction. Allergy to plastic eyeglass frames arises from sensitivities to the various chemicals used in the manufacturing process (Fig. 5.5).

MICROBIAL ALLERGY OF THE EYELIDS

Eczematoid Dermatitis Due to Microbial Allergy

Eczematoid dermatitis of the eyelids may arise on an allergic basis as a complication of bacterial, fungal, or other microorganismal infection present elsewhere.[2, 3] This basically allergic response to infectants must not be confused with the numerous types of dermatitis resulting from direct invasion of the skin of the eyelids by bacteria, viruses, and fungi. The types of dermatitis produced by invading microorganisms are entirely distinct and not germane to the subject. Allergic reactions of the eyelids due to bac-

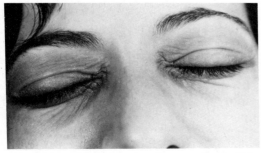

Figure 5.4 Allergy to fingernail polish. (Courtesy of Clay-Adams, Inc.)

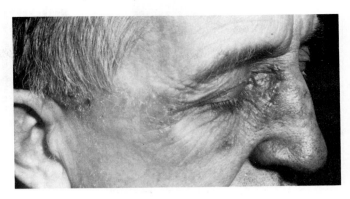

Figure 5.5 Contact allergy to plastic eyeglass frame. (Courtesy of New York Skin and Cancer Unit.)

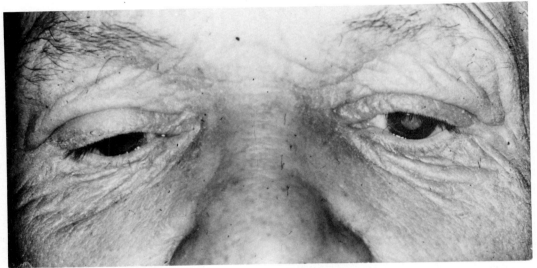

Figure 5.6 Atopic dermatitis of the eyelids. Note cataract left eye, a common occurrence in this condition. (Reprinted with permission from Theodore, F.H., and Schlossman, A. Ocular Allergy. Williams & Wilkins, Baltimore, 1958.)

teria generally are the result of neighboring infection of the adnexa, although rare syphilids and tuberculids need not follow this pattern. In fungal infections, however, the original focus may be far from the eye and entirely unrelated to it. In either event the eczema appears to be, in large measure, a manifestation of microbial allergy. While microbial dermatitis elsewhere on the body may result from a variety of infectants, including *Staphylococcus*, *Streptococcus*, and *Escherichia coli*, as far as the eyelids are concerned, the important bacterium involved is the *Staphylococcus*. On rare occasions streptococci are responsible. Eyelid eczema due to fungus sensitivity, an unusual occurrence to begin with, appears mainly as

trichophytids or moniliids. All types of infectious eczematoid reactions appear prone to secondary contact type allergies, especially from medicaments. Since the reverse also happens—that is, the secondary infection of primary allergic dermatitis—diagnostic problems may arise. However, fewer such differential difficulties should occur in regard to the eyelids, since the only type of infectious eczematoid reaction of practical importance encountered in this region, staphylococcal eczema, generally is associated with other ocular findings that afford valuable diagnostic clues.

Other diagnostic possibilities of chronic eyelid eczema besides infectious eczematoid staphylococcal dermatitis include

Table 5.2
Differential Diagnosis of Common Causes of Ocular Eczema[a]

	Contact Allergy	Staphylococcal Eczema	Atopic Dermatitis	Seborrheic Dermatitis
Personal and familial history of allergy	Not essential	Not essential	Usually positive for hay fever, asthma, urticaria, and other atopies	None
Other pertinent history	Recent exposure to allergenic substances	Previous staphylococcal infections	Previous infantile dermatitis; recurrences	Previous seborrhea
Bilaterality	Often unilateral	Often unilateral	Always bilateral	Almost always bilateral
Character of dermatitis	Moist, acute, or subacute with varying degrees of erythema, edema, and vesiculation	Moist, acute, or subacute with varying degrees of erythema, edema, and vesiculation	Dry, papular, and lichenified	Dry, erythematous nonvesicular, greasy scales
Associated dermatitis elsewhere	None	None	Antecubital, popliteal, sides and back of neck, mouth, and retroauricular	Scalp, forehead, eyebrows, nasolabial folds, retroauricular, presternal
Lid margins	Involved as part of process; not in itself distinctive	Ulcerative blepharitis and meibomitis present	Involved as part of the process; not in itself distinctive	Seborrheic squamous blepharitis
Conjunctiva	Usually not involved unless conjuctival contact occurred (contact dermatoconjunctivitis due to medicaments)	Definite, severe papillary conjunctivitis	Bilateral chronic papillary conjunctivitis	Usually not involved
Cornea	Rarely involved	Frequent involvement by superficial punctate keratitis of lower half of cornea (seen by slitlamp)	Rarely involved, but may be severe; peripheral or diffuse superficial areas with vascularization	No definite involvement
Cultures	Usually no significant growth	Toxigenic Staphylococcus grown from conjunctiva, lid margins, and meibomian secretion	Staphylococcus aureus (eyelids and conjunctiva) usually grown	No significant growth
Epithelial scrapings	Normal cytology	Cocci and neutrophiles on lid margins	Generally conjunctival eosinophilia of small degree	Budding yeast (Pityrosporum ovale) on lid margins
Intradermal tests	May be positive	Usually negative except for marked reaction to Staphylococcus toxoid	Few to many positives	Usually negative
Patch tests	Often positive	Negative	Negative	Negative
Treatment	Removal of cause; steroids	Antibacterial agents; toxoid and vaccine injections; steroids	Steroids; other nonspecific treatment; desensitization not especially helpful	Sulfur, mercury, other nonspecific agents

[a] Modified from Theodore and Schlossman.[1]

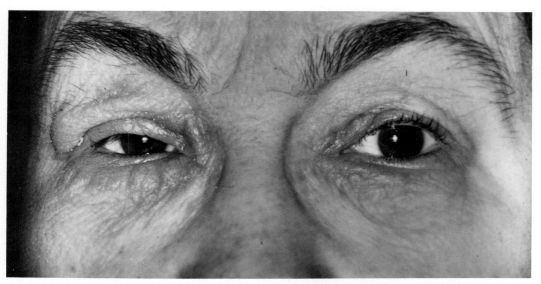

Figure 5.7 Staphylococcal eczema of the eyelids. (Reprinted with permission from Theodore, F.H. Differentiation and treatment of eczemas of the eyelids. Trans. Am. Acad. Ophthalmol. Otolaryngol. 58:708–723, 1954.)

Figure 5.8 Cultures of conjunctiva and eyelids (patient in Fig. 5.7) revealing numerous colonies of pathogenic *Staphylococcus aureus*; growth in form of "M" (*top left quadrant*) was obtained from expressed meibomian secretion. (Reprinted with permission from Theodore, F.H. Differentiation and treatment of eczemas of the eyelids. Trans. Am. Acad. Ophthalmol. Otolaryngol. 58:708–723, 1954.)

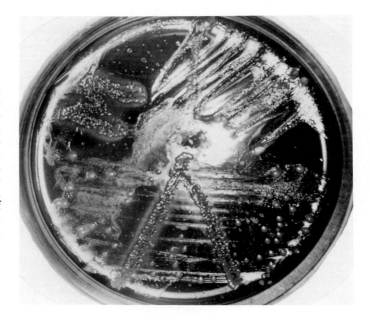

seborrheic or psoriatic eczema and atopic dermatitis (Fig. 5.6). These should always be considered before therapy is begun (Table 5.2).

Staphylococcal Eczema of the Eyelids

The importance of staphylococcal infections of the lid margin and conjunctiva as a major cause of eczema of the eyelids has not received the emphasis it deserves. While dermatitis actually is a relatively infrequent complication of such common infections, recent experience indicates that the condition is the most frequent cause of chronic eyelid eczema. Because its importance is not generally appreciated, it is often overlooked.

Many unrecognized, recurrent cases of

staphylococcal eczema of the eyelids are treated unsuccessfully for years as instances of contact allergy (Fig. 5.7). One cannot distinguish between the two conditions on the basis of the character of the dermatitis, since they look very much alike. What is required for the diagnosis and successful treatment of staphylococcal eczema is the demonstration that the focal point of the process is not the skin but instead the eye and its adnexa. When this is demonstrated and proper treatment instituted, the eczema, which is a secondary complication, gradually disappears. The key to diagnosis is routine detailed ophthalmological examination, both clinical and bacterial. This almost always will reveal the basis for the dermatitis, even if the primary focus is obscure, such as a minute abscess of a meibomian gland. The following findings differentiate staphylococcal eczema of the eyelids from the allergic variety: 1) blepharitis, with scaling and often ulcers of the eyelid margin; 2) meibomitis, either diffuse or focal; 3) superficial epithelial keratitis involving the inferior half of the cornea, readily seen on slitlamp examination after staining with fluorescein and considered as pathognomonic of staphylococcal con-

junctivitis; 4) strongly positive conjunctival and lid margin cultures, showing many toxin-producing staphylococci, often entirely out of numerical proportion to the objective clinical findings (Fig. 5.8); 5) absence of eosinophils in epithelial scrapings which, instead, usually reveal neutrophils and staphylococci, especially on the lid margins.

The immunopathogenesis of recurrent staphylococcal infection is unknown. A recent study has demonstrated IgE antibodies to *Staphylococcus aureus* in serum from patients with recurrent staphyloccal abscesses and chronic eczema. The formation of antistaphylococcal IgE may be relevant to the pathogenesis of staphyloccal infections. IgE mediates degranulation of basophils and mast cells and the released histamine has been shown to inhibit certain in vitro functions of polymorphonuclear leukocytes. Therefore, histamine may be interfering with the ability of polymorphonuclear leukocytes to effectively eliminate S. aureus.[4]

Treatment begins with adequate lid hygiene, often helped by topical application of 1% silver nitrate to the eyelid margins. Most valuable in the short run is the combined use of topical corticosteroids and

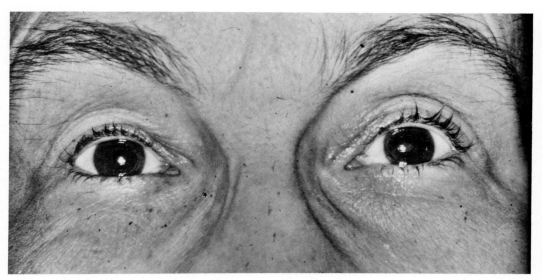

Figure 5.9 Complete cure of staphylococcal eczema (patient in Fig. 5.7). At this time bacterial cultures were negative. (Reprinted with permission from Theodore, F.H. Differentiation and treatment of eczemas of the eyelids. Trans. Am. Acad. Ophthalmol. Otolaryngol. 58:708–723, 1954.)

those anti-infective agents (antibiotics and sulfonamides) which the patient can tolerate. For long-term cure, desensitization with *Staphylococcus* toxoid and/or an autogenous vaccine obtained from the patient's conjunctiva and lid margins has been used (Fig. 5.9), with varying degrees of success. Unfortunately staphylococcus toxoid is no longer available.

Lid Margin Affections

In long-standing blepharitis, meibomitis, recurrent hordeola, and recurrent chalazia (all conditions in which staphylococcal infection plays an important role), secondary microbial allergy may supervene. Desensitization therapy may help in long-term treatment.

REFERENCES

1. Theodore, F.H., Schlossman, A. Ocular Allergy. Williams & Wilkins, Baltimore, 1958.
2. Theodore, F.H. Differentiation and treatment of eczemas of the eyelids. Trans. Am. Acad. Ophthalmol. Otolaryngol. 58:708–723, 1954.
3. Theodore, F.H. Staphylococcal eczema of the eyelids. Acta XVII Int. Congr. Ophthalmol. 2:609–615, 1955.
4. Schopfer, K., Baerlocher, K., Price, P., Krech, U., and Douglas, S.D. Staphylococcal IgE Antibodies, hyperimmunoglobulinemia E. and *Staphylococcus aureus* infections. N. Engl. J. Med. 300:835–837, 1979.

CHAPTER SIX

The Cornea

As with allergies of the conjunctiva, eyelids, and other parts of the eye, the various manifestations of corneal allergy are best understood when considered on the basis of the allergic mechanism involved. In fact, this mechanistic approach has particular advantages in regard to the cornea, because different types of allergy may give relatively similar clinical pictures, and because the type of reaction depends to a great extent on the degree of hypersensitivity, time of exposure, and other factors which alter the clinical picture. A classification of corneal immune reactions is presented in Table 6.1.

ATOPIC REACTIONS OF THE CORNEA

The absence of mast cells and the limited opportunity for blood-borne basophils to enter the cornea means that IgE-mediated reactions are probably rare, secondary to those occurring in the adjacent conjunctiva, or mild, because of the lack of mediators.

Atopic reactions of the cornea are most commonly caused by pollen allergy or by certain ingestants.[1,2] They are mainly superficial in nature, although occasionally deep keratitis does occur. Superficial keratitis due to atopy is much more common than the literature would seem to indicate. It consists of diffuse or patchy superficial punctate staining with fluorescein. Because of the mildness of atopic corneal reactions, most patients are not referred to the ophthalmologist. In other patients, the diagnosis may be missed by allergists who have no experience in the use of the slitlamp. Also, many atopic reactions are self-limited or improve as a result of the treatment of the general atopy.

Corneal Reactions to Pollens and Dusts

While the conjunctiva is commonly affected by hay fever, corneal involvement is much less frequent and occurs only in more severe cases. It is generally confined to superficial keratitis with a few isolated areas that stain with fluorescein. We have also noted mild keratitis in conjunctival tests utilizing pollen extract. Such keratitis is often self-limited and responds readily to the same treatment as the conjunctivitis. This mild lesion presents no problem either diagnostically or therapeutically and is of little cause for concern. More severe reactions may occur from other pollens, such as corn and orris root. In severe generalized hypersensitivity to dusts, the cornea may become involved.

Corneal Reactions to Ingestants

Corneal allergies due to foods are generally more severe than those due to inhalants. While they may at times be superficial, the allergies tend to involve the corneal stroma. Foods that have been incriminated include cottonseed meal, wheat, strawberries, cucumbers, cheese, cola, egg white, chocolate, rye, and nuts. In addition, corneal allergy has been reported from the internal use of a mixture containing phenacetin and antipyrine.

CONTACT ALLERGY OF THE CORNEA

The cornea is often involved in contact allergies of the eye. This is usually part of a contact dermatoconjunctivitis, so that the involvement of these tissues points to the correct diagnosis. Since the cornea may show only mild superficial keratitis, with diffuse or patchy superficial punctate staining with fluorescein, its involvement may be easily overlooked when other parts of the eye have a more marked

Table 6.1
Clinical Reactions of the Cornea

1. Atopic allergy (immediate)
   a. Topical allergens: superficial keratitis (rarely ulceration)
   b. Generalized allergy: superficial and marginal keratitis (rarely deep)
2. Contact allergy (delayed)
   a. Drugs: superficial keratitis; deep ulcerations
   b. Other contactants: superficial keratitis, deep keratitis
3. Microbial allergy
   a. Syphilis, tubercle bacilli (other bacteria): interstitial keratitis
   b. Tubercle bacilli, staphylococci, other bacteria, coccidioides immitis, nematodes: phlyctenulosis
   c. Staphylococci: catarrhal ulcers and infiltrates
   d. Virus of herpes simplex: disciform keratitis
   e. Adenoviruses: subepithelial opacities
4. Keratitis of possible immune origin
   a. Vernal conjunctivitis
   b. Atopic dermatitis
   c. Rosacea
   d. Immune reactions from contact lenses
5. Peripheral corneal ulcers
   a. Mooren's ulcer
   b. Peripheral ulcers associated with systemic diseases
6. Corneal transplants (delayed)

reaction. In some instances, the lids and conjunctiva are slightly affected but the keratitis is extremely severe. On occasion, the superficial cornea may show a similar picture to that of atopic allergic keratitis, and differential diagnosis will then depend on history and elimination of the offending allergen.

Often, however, corneal involvement may dominate the scene. Severe contact keratitis may extend into the deeper layers of the cornea and may be accompanied by iritis. Occasionally, the process is essentially subepithelial, with no staining of the cornea.

The responsible allergens include a variety of ophthalmic medicaments, such as local anesthetics, mydriatic alkaloids, antibiotics, sulfonamides, mercurials, quaternary ammonium compounds, lanolin, coal tar dyes, orris root, and vegetable products.

Special emphasis must be given to possibly severe reactions to some of the newer and better local anesthetics, such as proparacaine (Ophthaine, Ophthetic), and to a lesser degree, benoxinate hydrochloride (Dorsacaine) (Fig. 6.1). Theodore[3] has reported a number of instances of bilateral necrotizing epithelial reactions which, in some cases, required the patient's hospitalization because of severe disability due to pain and poor vision after the instillation of a single drop. Fortunately, using steroids, recovery was complete in patients with these acute idiosyncrasies. However, the constant home use of such anesthetics for chronic eye con-

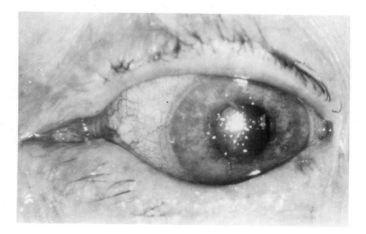

Figure 6.1 Idiosyncratic corneal reaction to proparacaine (Ophthaine). Marked epithelial necrosis with multiple small filaments occurring 25 minutes after instillation of the anesthetic drops. No dermatoconjunctivitis.

ditions may cause severe, deeper corneal allergies or toxic reactions that may result in permanent disabilities and visual loss.

MICROBIALLERGIC KERATITIS

Allergic reactions of the cornea to products of bacteria, protozoa, fungi, helminths, and other similar protein products give a wide variety of corneal lesions. It is interesting that certain bacteria have long been associated with certain specific corneal changes. Thus, the classical picture of interstitial keratitis was attributed to syphilis and phlyctenular keratoconjunctivitis was most commonly traced to the allergenic products of the tubercle bacillus, especially in those parts of the world where tuberculosis is still a common disease. Actually, in the United States, except for Alaskan Eskimos and American Indians, staphylococcal antigens are probably the most common cause of phlyctenulosis.

Interstitial Keratitis

Interstitial keratitis denotes an inflammation of the corneal stroma not primarily involving the anterior or posterior surfaces.[4] There is an invasion of the corneal stroma by inflammatory cells and then vessels. An allergic mechanism appears to offer the best explanation for the two major types of interstitial keratitis encountered clinically, syphilitic and tubercular. Syphilitic interstitial keratitis is the most common type of interstitial keratitis. In the majority of cases the disease is congenital. Syphilitic interstitial keratitis particularly involves the deeper layers of the cornea and is associated with an anterior uveitis with keratic precipitates. The residual corneal changes include stromal opacities and blood vessels. As a late manifestation of hereditary syphilis, interstitial keratitis is usually bilateral. In acquired syphilis, most cases are unilateral.

Evidence for an allergic etiology is based on 1) ineffectiveness of specific antisyphilitic therapy, 2) effectiveness of corticosteroids, and 3) rare onset of interstitial keratitis during the course of systemic arsenic therapy. The treatment of syphilitic interstitial keratitis includes topical cycloplegics and corticosteroids.

Tuberculous interstitial keratitis is often unilateral, involves the middle or deeper layers of the cornea, and is frequently limited to a sector usually only in the inferior cornea. The treatment of tuberculous interstitial keratitis includes treatment of the general disease with antibiotics and the use of topical corticosteroids and cycloplegics.

A diffuse interstitial keratitis has also been described in association with viral infections such as mumps, herpes, and influenza. Diffuse interstitial keratitis can rarely be seen as a complication of trypanosomiasis. Nonsyphilitic interstitial keratitis associated with vestibuloauditory symptoms was described by Cogan.[5] Interstitial keratitis with no proven etiology or association has been found by the authors to respond dramatically to topical corticosteroids (Fig. 6.2).

Phlyctenulosis

Phlyctenular keratoconjunctivitis is characterized by nodules of the conjunctiva and cornea occurring mainly in children.[6,7] These nodules appear first at the limbus then spread to the bulbar conjunctiva and cornea. The lesions last approximately 10 days to 2 weeks. The phlyctenule occasionally resolves spontaneously but usually undergoes necrosis with sloughing of the overlying epithelium and formation of an ulcer (Fig. 6.3).

Phlyctenular ulcers of the cornea may appear as marginal ulcers. These marginal ulcers differ from catarrhal ulcers in that they leave no clear space between the ulcer and the limbus and their axes are frequently perpendicular rather than parallel to the circumference of the cornea. The marginal ulcers may remain stationary but may also spread centrally as a fascicular ulcer or wandering phlyctenule, which is perhaps the most characteristic of all the phlyctenular corneal lesions. The peripheral area of the ulcer may heal while the central margin remains active and progresses across the cornea preceded by gray infiltration. Vessels run in a straight course from the limbus and follow the ulcer centrally. Scars are formed

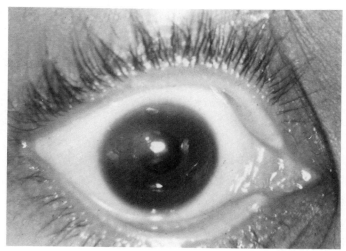

Figure 6.2 Nonluetic interstitial keratitis involving upper temporal cornea. Dramatic clearing with topical steroids.

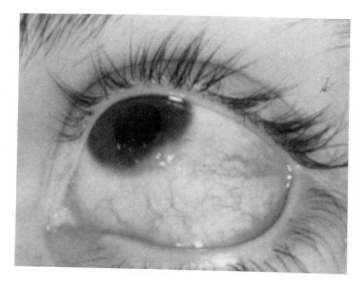

Figure 6.3 Phlyctenular keratoconjunctivitis in patient strongly positive to tuberculin. Rapid cure with topical cortisone. (Reprinted with permission from Theodore, F.H., and Schlossman, A. Ocular Allergy. Williams & Wilkins, Baltimore, 1958.)

only on the cornea and are triangular with the base at the limbus. A rarely seen type of corneal involvement is miliary phlyctenulosis, in which there are minute phlyctenules that cover the corneal surface. Other manifestations of corneal phlyctenulosis include superficial and deep diffuse central infiltrates without ulceration, seen most commonly in recurrent phlyctenulosis of long duration and phlyctenular pannus that is characteristically irregular and inferior in location.

Phlyctenules are subepithelial inflammatory nodules composed of leukocytes and blood vessels. The inflammatory cells include macrophages, lymphocytes, plasma cells, and polymorphonuclear leukocytes. The nodule may resolve or ulcerate.

Phlyctenulosis has been related to tuberculosis in the Eskimo and Indian populations in the United States. It has been suggested that the eye is sensitive to tuberculoprotein at an early age and that an attack of phlyctenulosis is precipitated by the presentation of tuberculoprotein to the sensitized eye either by the blood stream or by inoculation into the conjunctival sac. Spontaneous desensitization seems to occur in adult life. Vitamin deficiency, malnutrition, blepharitis, and acute bacterial conjunctivitis contribute to the disease and may act as trigger mechanisms.

At present most cases of phlyctenulosis are being related to staphylococcal blepharitis. Photophobia and tearing are less severe and corneal perforations are rarer in phlyctenular disease associated with staphylococci than in phlyctenular disease associated with tuberculosis. Phlyctenulosis has also been related to *Candida albicans*, *Coccidioides immitis*, the agent of lymphogranuloma venereum, and nematodes.

Topical corticosteroids adequately control phlyctenular keratoconjunctivitis. Systemic and subconjunctival corticosteroids are generally not necessary. Any secondary bacterial infections should be treated with antibiotics. An associated staphylococcal blepharitis should be controlled with lid scrubs followed by antibiotic ointment. Cycloplegics should be used when the cornea is involved.

Phlyctenules have been studied experimentally since the turn of the century. The production of phlyctenules has been reported after the instillation of tuberculin into the conjunctival sac of tuberculous rabbits[8] and after the instillation of staphylococci into the conjunctival sac of rabbits sensitized to this organism.[9] In 1962, it was stated that experimental results of phlyctenule production reported to that time were unconvincing and without histopathological documentation and that a true experimental model did not exist.[10] In 1972, experimental attempts that failed to produce phlyctenules in rabbits and guinea pigs were reported and a plea was made for communications setting forth detailed methodology for the production of phlyctenules in animals because reports in the literature lacked sufficient and perhaps essential details.[11]

A rabbit model of phlyctenulosis and catarrhal infiltrates has recently been developed.[12] Rabbits immunized and boosted with phenol-inactivated *Staphylococcus aureus* showed a fourfold or greater increase in antibody titer and delayed hypersensitivity to *S. aureus*. After topical challenge with viable *S. aureus*, the rabbits in this model developed vascularized, elevated nodular infiltrates of the cornea resembling phlyctenules in humans and peripheral corneal infiltrates running parallel to the limbus and separated from it by a lucid interval resembling catarrhal infiltrates in humans. The nodular corneal infiltrates were found in a subepithelial location and were composed of vessels, polymorphonuclear leukocytes, and mononuclear cells including lymphocytes, plasma cells, and macrophages. The peripheral corneal infiltrates separated from the limbus by a lucid interval were found in the anterior stroma beneath the corneal epithelium and were composed of polymorphonuclear leukocytes and mononuclear cells (Fig. 6.4).

Catarrhal Ulcers and Infiltrates

The catarrhal infiltrate and ulcer is usually a complication of long-standing staphylococcal blepharitis and conjunc-

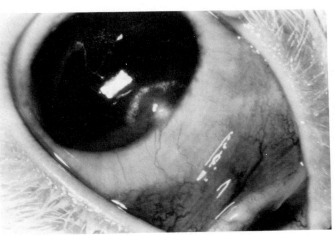

Figure 6.4 Elevated vascularized nodular infiltrate of rabbit cornea resembling human phlyctenule. Incomplete ring infiltrate central to nodule.

tivitis.[13,14] Cultures of the lid margins usually yield many colonies of mannitol-positive, coagulase-positive S. *aureus* or, in rare instances, coagulase-positive *Staphylococcus albus*.[13]

Catarrhal ulcers are common in adults and rare in children. A distinct lucid interval separates the peripheral corneal infiltrates and ulcers from the corneoscleral limbus. The direction of spread of the corneal ulcers is concentric with the corneoscleral limbus, with no tendency to spread centrally. The infiltrate appears first and is followed by fluorescein staining of the surface as ulceration develops, unlike peripheral herpetic keratitis which begins with an epithelial defect that is followed by an infiltrate. Sensation is normal or very slightly diminished over these areas. Blood vessels may eventually bridge the lucid interval, and after healing there may be a peripheral pannus directed to the ulcer site. The ulcer shows a marked tendency to recur. There are reports of these marginal ulcers coalescing to form ring ulcers[14] (Figs. 6.5–6.7).

Gram and Giemsa stains of corneal scrapings reveal polymorphonuclear leukocytes, but no bacteria. Corneal cultures are negative for bacteria. The lesion is thought to represent an antigen-antibody reaction with complement activation and polymorphonuclear infiltration in patients sensitized to staphylococcal antigens.[15] In fact, antibody and C3 complement have been demonstrated in the ca-

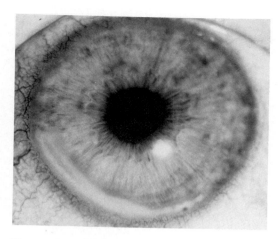

Figure 6.6 Coalescence of catarrhal infiltrates forming a ring segment.

tarrhal ulcer.[16] A rabbit model of catarrhal infiltrates has been developed.[12]

Although marginal or catarrhal ulcers are associated with staphylococcal conjunctivitis or blepharitis in the overwhelming majority of cases, they have also been found in association with positive conjunctival cultures for the diplobacillus of Morax-Axenfeld and Koch-Weeks bacillus.[15] Catarrhal ulcers have been reported recently in association with acute beta hemolytic streptococcal conjunctivitis and chronic dacryocystitis (lacrimal conjunctivitis of Morax).[17] Marginal catarrhal ulcers may also occur on a primary ocular basis in the absence of conjunctival or eyelid infection or demonstrable systemic disease.

TREATMENT

Basically catarrhal ulcers and infiltrates clear promptly with adequate treatment of the conjunctival infection if one exists. If such proper anti-infectious agents are combined with a corticosteroid, healing is dramatic and represents one of the prime indications for the use of antibiotic-steroid or sulfa-steroid mixtures in ophthalmic practice. Steroids are even more necessary in those cases where infection does not appear to be present.

Prevention of recurrences in the absence of a known etiology is difficult. However, in those patients where a microbiallergic reaction to chronic staphy-

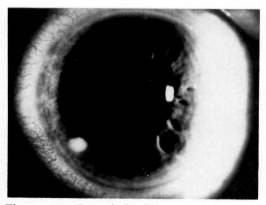

Figure 6.5 Catarrhal infiltrate and ulcer at 8 o'clock position with lucid interval separating it from limbus.

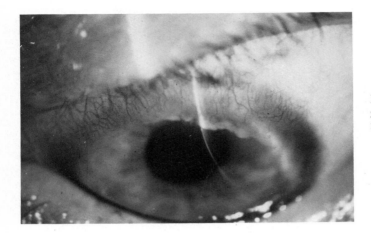

Figure 6.7 Confluent marginal ulcers with pannus formation.

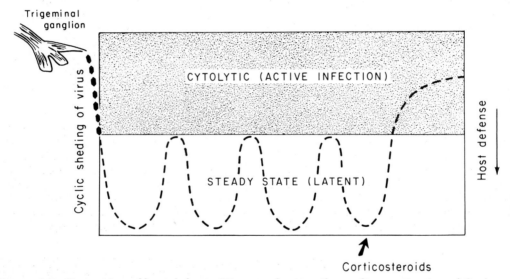

Figure 6.8 Depression of host defense. Diagram showing the cyclic reactivation of the herpes simplex virus from its latent state in the trigeminal ganglion. Clinically active disease probably results from a combination or reactivation of the virus and a depression of the host defense from use of, for example, corticosteroids.

lococcal infection appears to the cause, a regime including topical antibacterial agents, lid margin treatments such as "scrubs" with Johnson and Johnson's baby shampoo or 1% silver nitrate applied with a cotton tipped applicator may eliminate or reduce staphylococcal counts. In addition to such regular treatments, desensitization with staphylococcal vaccines and, in the past, *Staphylococcus* toxoid, have proved successful in prevention of recurrences.

Disciform Keratitis

Seroepidemiological studies show that over 70% of the population has had some exposure to herpes simplex, either as a clinical or subclinical infection.[18] Considering how widespread this virus is, it is postulated that an immune imbalance in the host may be required to result in activation of the virus and subsequent disease. It is also possible that different clinical patterns of herpetic ocular disease may be attributed to differing biological behavior or virulence of specific stains of herpes simplex virus.[19] An active infectious dendritic keratitis is often associated with a history of depression in the host defense, either in a healthy patient or in patients immunosuppressed by an underlying disease or iatrogenically by a systemic immunosuppressive agent[20] (Fig. 6.8). In otherwise healthy patients, one can often elicit a history of stress due to such things as psychogenic causes, fevers, sunburn, and menstruation. This presumably raises endogenous levels of 17-hydroxycorticosteroids and results in some depression of the host defense. Iatrogenic immunosuppression with systemic corticosteroids, also results in an active, infectious keratitis characterized by multiple large dendrites (Fig. 6.9).

Once activated, the viral antigen causes an immune response by the host to clear the virus. Immune responses can then result in further damage on an immunogenic basis.

If the virus enters the stroma, the immune response called upon to get rid of the virus can cause reactions which result in severe stromal ulceration and inflammation, clinically known as necrotizing stromal disease or interstitial keratitis.[21] This interplay of ongoing viral replication and a continuing host immune response has been shown to lead to both an immune complex (type III) and the more important cell-mediated (type IV) immunopathology.

Herpes disciform keratitis is another form of stromal disease with an immune basis. It is thought that viral antigen becomes integrated into the stromal fibroblast, thereby changing its antigenic character. The body no longer recognizes the cells as "self" and mounts a cell-mediated immune response, manifesting itself clinically as disciform corneal edema.[22]

Disciform keratitis may be caused by organisms other than herpes simplex, such as the viruses responsible for mumps, infectious mononucleosis, herpes zoster, and vaccinia. In the absence of a preceding history of a dendritic figure, it may be hard to conclude that the disciform edema is due to herpes simplex. In addition, edema may involve the entire cornea, not only a central disc-shaped area (Fig. 6.10).

Originally, disciform keratitis was used to describe a disc-like opacity situated in the corneal stroma, often assuming twice its usual thickness in the involved area and associated with "descemetitis." Usually the corneal epithelium was relatively intact, and staining with fluorescein revealed little or nothing. Most such cases were attributed to herpes simplex infec-

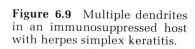
Figure 6.9 Multiple dendrites in an immunosuppressed host with herpes simplex keratitis.

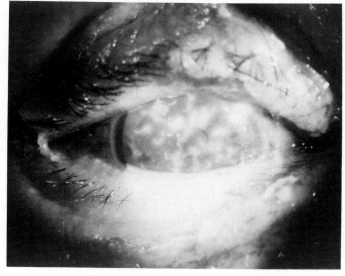

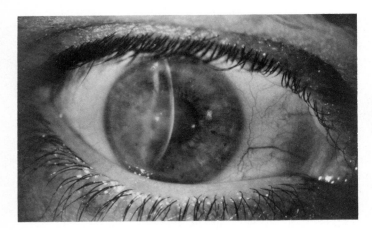

Figure 6.10 Disciform keratitis in a patient with herpes simplex.

tion, and it was hypothesized that the virus had somehow entered the stroma through the epithelium. Many times the so-called point of entrance could not be demonstrated. Such cases were in themselves very serious. Resultant central opacities, after the edema of the cornea had subsided, could reduce vision to the extent of industrial blindness. There seems no clear-cut evidence, other than circumstantial, that the condition is always due to herpes simplex. Sometimes herpes zoster and vaccinia seem causative. In still other instances the cause is not demonstrable.

Disciform keratitis responds well to low doses of corticosteroids, but their usage is a matter of clinical judgment in each case because of the potential side effects of steroids. In summary, an immune imbalance may occur in various stages of herpes simplex keratitis. The depression of the host defense can lead to an acute infection. The host's attempted control of virus antigen can then result in an inflammatory disease against the virus itself or against the cornea if the virus becomes integrated into the corneal fibroblast.

Adenovirus Keratitis

A microbiallergic basis for the subepithelial opacities occurring in adenovirus type 8 (epidemic keratoconjunctivitis, EKC) appears to be a strong possibility. Theodore has observed many patients in whom the opacities (which occur at a time when infectivity is over) clear dramatically with the use of topical steroids, only

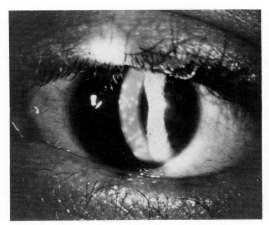

Figure 6.11 Discrete subepithelial infiltrates in a patient with epidemic keratoconjunctivitis (EKC).

to reappear when the medicament is discontinued. Some of these patients receiving steroids show recurrence of opacities as long as 2 years after the original epidemic keratoconjunctivitis infection if the drug is stopped completely. So, in order to avoid a form of steroid "addiction," we do not advocate their use unless central opacities seriously bother the patient, either subjectively or visually (Fig. 6.11). It has recently been shown that these lesions in EKC consist of clusters of lymphocytes.[23]

SUPERFICIAL PUNCTATE KERATITIS (THYGESON)

Thygeson's superficial punctate keratitis (SPK) is another disease entity, possibly with an immune basis, since it responds so exquisitely to steroids. It usually occurs in a white or only slightly inflamed eye and the patient has symptoms of foreign body sensation or light sensitivity. It is most common in young males. The lesions occur as clusters made of tiny elevated dots and may remind the observer of the magnified appearance of snowflakes. These usually stain with fluorescein (Fig. 6.12).

KERATITIS IN VERNAL CONJUNCTIVITIS

The various corneal manifestations of vernal conjunctivitis, a disease apparently related to atopic dermatitis, have been described under conjunctival allergic reactions. Their occasional severe nature and sequelae have been emphasized. Keratoconus is associated with vernal conjunctivitis.

KERATITIS ASSOCIATED WITH ATOPIC DERMATITIS

Corneal involvement of varying intensity may complicate chronic atopic dermatitis. According to Hogan,[24] the corneal affection may occur simultaneously with, or following repeated exacerbations of conjunctivitis. The superficial third of the periphery of the cornea is affected first (Fig. 6.13). The corneal stroma near Bowman's membrane becomes clouded. The lesion gradually spreads deeper into the stroma, and after some time, blood vessels push in from the limbus. The corneal

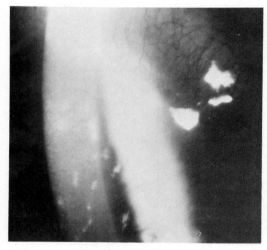

Figure 6.12 Thygeson's superficial punctate keratitis (SPK) consisting of lesions occurring as clusters of tiny, sometimes elevated dots in a relatively quiet eye.

Figure 6.13 Keratitis associated with atopic dermatitis (drawing). (Courtesy of Dr. M. J. Hogan.)

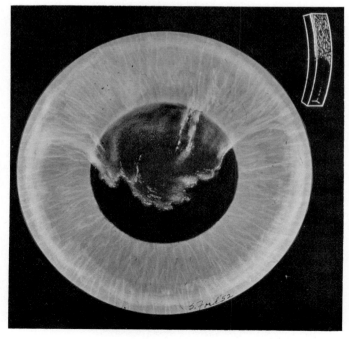

epithelium covering the area of keratitis become edematous and shows minute punctate staining with fluorescein. In some instances, the entire corneal becomes hazy and vascularized, resulting in diminished visual acuity. Steroid therapy, both local and systemic, is the most effective medicament. At times keratoconus is associated with atopic dermatitis.

KERATOCONUS

Keratoconus is associated with allergic diseases such as vernal conjunctivitis and atopic conditions. Serum IgE levels have been found to be raised in keratoconus, markedly in those cases associated with atopic diseases.[25] Moreover, patients with this corneal condition may manifest severe and extensive dermatitis with lichenification and pigmentation, severe bronchial asthma, and reactions to food and inhalant allergens.

ROSACEA KERATITIS

In our experience the unrecognized presence of early rosacea causing resistant blepharoconjunctivitis, and later keratitis, is very common. Rosacea is a chronic hyperemic disease of the skin classically affecting the nose, forehead, and cheeks. It is characterized by erythema, telangiectasia, papules, pustules, and hypertrophic sebaceous glands. The most advanced

form of the disease is rhinophyma. The ocular manifestations involve the lids, conjunctiva, and cornea. They include blepharitis, meibomitis, chalazia, styes, and diffuse hyperemic conjunctiva. In our studies of early ocular rosacea we have been particularly impressed with the value of the consistent finding of diffuse vascularization of the lid margins (seen with the biomicroscope) as one of the most valuable early diagnostic clues.

Usually the keratitis in rosacea is located in the lower two-thirds of the cornea; on rare occasions the upper cornea is involved. Superficial epithelial pannus due to peripheral vascularization with peripheral superficial corneal infiltration is first noted, an extension of the conjunctival process. Later, the subepithelial infiltrates form a typically triangular tongue-like shape and progress towards the center of the cornea. Corneal erosions and frank ulcerations develop with increased superficial vascularization of the cornea (Fig. 6.14). Recurrent ulcerations give the cornea an irregular surface, while thinning leads to facet formation. Symptomatology is severe, with complaints of burning, tearing and foreign body sensation. The etiology is unclear, but an immune mechanism is suggested, with a possible relationship to staphylococcal allergy.

Until the advent of corticosteroids, therapy was usually ineffectual; steroids

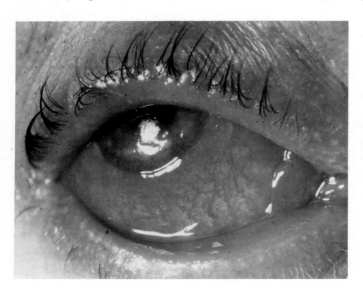

Figure 6.14 Rosacea keratoconjunctivitis. (Reprinted with permission from Theodore, F. H., and Schlossman, A. Ocular Allergy. Williams & Wilkins, Baltimore, 1958.)

are beneficial both systemically and topically. In the past 10 years, systemic tetracycline has been used successfully for many resistant cases, ever since this method was introduced in the field of dermatology. When tetracycline is not tolerated, erythromycin is sometimes effective. This specific approach has been well-documented in recent ophthalmic literature by Brown.[26, 27] The exact etiology of rosacea remains obscure.

CORNEAL INFILTRATES ASSOCIATED WITH THE USE OF CONTACT LENSES

In a series of 278 patients fitted with therapeutic soft hydrophilic contact lenses on an extended wear basis, 11 patients developed stromal infiltrates.[28] Seven had small, multiple grayish corneal infiltrates that were not thought to be typical bacterial or fungal infections and disappeared on discontinuation of use of the lenses. In four cases the corneal lesions appeared as dense, round, yellowish-white infiltrates that had a stormy course that responded to antibiotics. They were thought to be typical bacterial infections and resulted in permanent corneal scarring. Bacterial corneal ulcers are a threat to cosmetic soft contact lens wearers, and it has been shown that a substantial percentage of soft lens wearers are inadequately disinfecting their lenses.[29]

Subepithelial infiltrates in soft contact lens wearers have been attributed to chlamydial infections.[30] It is believed that chlamydial keratoconjunctivitis may be completely asymptomatic and become apparent when soft contact lenses are worn.

Corneal infiltrates resembling catarrhal infiltrates have been noted in soft contact lens wearers.[31] They have been attributed to an immunological reaction to staphylococcal antigens because the infiltrates disappeared if staphylococci were eliminated from the eyelids. Anoxia may also be a factor, since fitting a flatter lens also alleviated the problem (Fig. 6.15).

Anterior stromal infiltrates of the cornea have also been shown to be a manifestation of delayed hypersensitivity to thimerosal.[32] In this study, the conjunctival hyperemia and corneal infiltrates re-

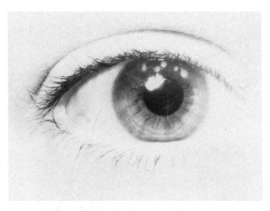

Figure 6.15 Discrete peripheral corneal infiltrations of the superficial stroma after soft contact lens wear. (Courtesy of Dr. T. C. Spoor.)

solved after discontinuation of soft contact lenses but reappeared when chemically disinfected soft contact lenses were placed in the eye. Moreover, while using heat disinfection and saline without preservatives, all patients were able to wear their soft contact lenses without symptoms and signs of inflammation. Bacterial cultures of the conjunctiva, lids, lens cases, lens solutions, and eye cosmetics were not helpful in these cases. Conjunctival cultures for adenovirus and Chlamydial titers were negative. Giemsa stain of conjunctival scrapings showed a few mononuclear leukocytes and rare eosinophils but no inclusion bodies. Occlusive patch tests and intradermal tests showed positive delayed hypersensitivity reactions to the chemical disinfectants. Occlusive patch tests with thimerosal suggested that this preservative was responsible for the conjunctival and corneal reactions (Figs. 6.16 and 6.17).

Another study described patients with redness, irritation, and corneal changes related to soft contact lens wear and also suggested that this represented a hypersensitivity to thimerosal with the thiosalicylate moiety being the culprit.[33]

MOOREN'S ULCER

Mooren's ulcer is a chronic, painful ulceration of the cornea which begins in the periphery with a steep, undermined, and occasionally infiltrated leading border.

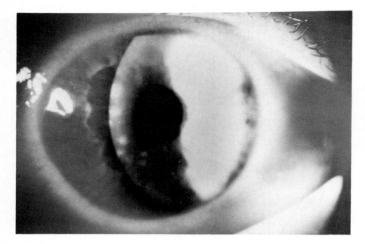

Figure 6.16 Anterior stromal infiltrates of cornea in soft contact lens wearer. Positive intradermal and occlusive patch tests to thimerosal.

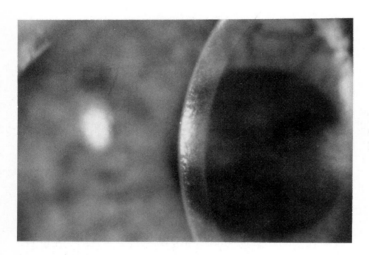

Figure 6.17 Anterior location of infiltrates demonstrated in patient shown in Fig. 6.17.

The ulcer advances centripetally and circumferentially, leaving in its wake a thinned, vascularized cornea. It is a rare disease, with most patients being affected in the fourth to sixth decade.[34] It is bilateral in approximately 25% of cases but does not necessarily develop simultaneously in both eyes.[35] An interval of several years may lapse between the involvement of the first eye and the second.

Mooren's ulcer may begin as one or two patches of gray infiltrate near the margin of the cornea which slowly spread, coalesce, and eventually break down to form a shallow furrow.[36, 37] The ulcer spreads slowly, undermining the corneal epithelium and the superficial lamellae at its advancing border so that a gray, infiltrated, overhanging edge is formed, which in some cases can be lifted up.[35] This is characteristic of Mooren's ulcer. There is usually some swelling and hyperemia of the limbus adjacent to the ulcer. The ulcer may spread slowly and remorselessly or may be self-limited. In some cases remissions and exacerbations are common.

The spread of the corneal ulcer occurs in three directions: around the periphery, toward the center of the cornea, and occasionally into the sclera. Behind the actively progressing edge of the ulcer, healing takes place from the periphery with the development of new vessels, but the healed area remains permanently clouded with poor visual acuity.[35] In some cases all that is eventually left is Descemet's membrane and the most posterior corneal lamellae, covered by conjunctival epithelium. There is little tendency for fibrous tissue formation as a reparative response (Figs. 6.18 and 6.19).

A mild iritis is found, and a secondary cataract may develop, but hypopyon or perforation rarely occur.[35, 37]

During the stages of advancing disease, the patients usually experience severe pain, photophobia, and lacrimation. Visual acuity is decreased because of extension of the ulcer into the pupillary area or because of the development of irregular astigmatism.

In 1971, Wood and Kaufman[38] suggested that there were two different types of Mooren's ulcer: 1) a unilateral limited type, occurring in older patients and responding to relatively conservative surgery after one or two operative procedures and 2) a relentlessly progressive type occurring most commonly in younger patients, frequently involving the sclera as well as the peripheral cornea and not responding to any therapy.

Histopathological examination of the conjunctiva adjacent to Mooren's ulcer shows plasma cells and lymphocytes with an occasional polymorphonuclear leukocyte.[39] The leading edge of the ulcer is infiltrated with leukocytes.[40] In the ulcerated area, Bowman's membrane, as well as the corneal stroma is destroyed, except for the most posterior lamellae.[35] Descemet's membrane and the endothelium are not damaged.

An unequivocal etiology has not been established for Mooren's ulcer. It has been related to previous ocular trauma, with

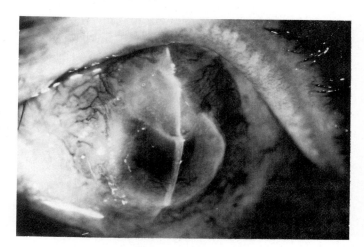

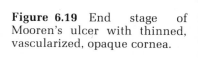

Figure 6.18 Mooren's ulcer with steep central border indicated by slit-beam.

Figure 6.19 End stage of Mooren's ulcer with thinned, vascularized, opaque cornea.

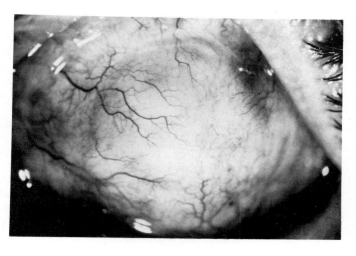

many cases having either physical or chemical injuries antedating the development of the ulcer.[38] Mooren-like ulcers have been reported following intracapsular cataract extractions[41] and also following herpes zoster ophthalmicus.[42] Bacteria and viruses have been postulated but never proven as causes.[36] Mooren's ulcer has been related to metabolic disorders and malnutrition, trophic disturbances involving the trigeminal nerve, deficiency of vitamin B1, and ankylostomiasis.[35–37] Primary ischemic necrosis of limbal vessels has been postulated as being important in the development of these ulcers.[50] The conjunctiva adjacent to Mooren's ulcer has been shown to produce collagenase and proteoglycanase, both of which may be important in corneal ulceration.[39]

In recent years an autoimmune etiology has been suggested for Mooren's ulcer because of the demonstration of plasma cells in the conjunctiva adjacent to the ulcer,[39] the finding of immunoglobulins and complement bound to the conjunctival epithelium and basement membrane adjacent to the ulcer,[44–46] the presence of circulating antibodies to conjunctival and corneal epithelium,[44,45] and the demonstration that the lymphocytes of patients with Mooren's ulcer are sensitized to corneal antigen.[47] It may be that Mooren's ulcer represents a final common pathway to a variety of insults to the cornea in susceptible patients. The corneal tissue may be altered in such a way that autoimmune phenomena develop that are either intimately involved in the pathogenesis of the ulcer or are responsible for aggravating and perpetuating the basic disease process, whatever it may be.

Treatment with subconjunctival injections of heparin adjacent to the ulcer have been recommended to improve the primary ischemic process that has been postulated to exist in this condition,[43] but their value is controversial. Collagenase inhibitors applied topically and systemic corticosteroids are ineffective. Soft contact lenses may relieve pain but probably have little effect on the ulcerative process.[34]

The limited, unilateral form of Mooren's ulcer may respond to topical corticosteroids in some cases. If unsuccessful, a resection of 3 to 4 mm of the conjunctiva adjacent to the ulcer may be tried.[48] This is generally successful in the limited, unilateral variety of Mooren's ulcer but may have to be repeated. Because the adjacent conjunctiva produces proteoglycanase and collagenase and contains plasma cells that may be producing autoantibodies,[39] its excision may facilitate healing.

There is no consistently effective treatment for the bilateral, relentlessly progressive type of Mooren's ulcer. Topical steroids are generally unsuccessful. It may be necessary to repeatedly resect the conjunctiva adjacent to the ulcer, and this may prove temporarily successful.[48] Lamellar and penetrating keratoplasties performed in a setting of acute disease activity are uniformly unsuccessful and may be invaded by the disease process. Following destruction of all but the posterior corneal lamellae, ulceration and the associated inflammatory activity subside. This end stage of Mooren's ulcer may be hastened by lamellar keratectomy of the remaining central island of cornea as suggested by Maumenee.[49] The epithelium rapidly heals over the area of the excised corneal tissue with subsidence of ulceration, inflammation, and pain. When these eyes have been quiet for several months, penetrating keratoplasty may be successful and may provide useful vision.[50]

PERIPHERAL CORNEAL ULCERS ASSOCIATED WITH SYSTEMIC DISEASES

Ring infiltrates and ulcers have been associated with systemic diseases that include bacillary dysentery, influenza, acute leukemia, periarteritis nodosa, scleroderma, and lupus erythematosus.[15,51] The infiltrate and eventually the ulcer form a continuous ring in the periphery of the cornea. The ring infiltrate is usually continuous from the onset but sometimes develops as a coalescence of multiple discrete infiltrates that appear near the limbus. The coalescence of these discrete infiltrates to form a continuous ring may take a few days to a week, unlike Mooren's ulcer, which takes several months to surround the cornea. Unlike catarrhal ulcers where the conjunctival reaction is

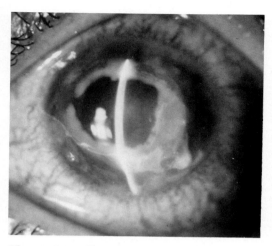

Figure 6.20 Dramatic onset of ring ulcer (occurring in 24 hours) in a patient with a past history of multiple small peripheral marginal ulcers. Rapid and complete clearing with topical and systemic corticosteroids.

generalized, the conjunctival reaction associated with ring ulcers is minimal except for the circumcorneal hyperemia. Catarrhal ulcers are usually unilateral, while ring ulcers are generally bilateral. In patients with ring ulcers, cultures of the conjunctiva are generally negative for pathogenic organisms. Topical corticosteroids have been used to treat ring infiltrates and ulcers[51] (Fig. 6.20).

Wegener's granulomatosis and periarteritis nodosa may be associated with marginal corneal ulcers, with features that resemble early stages of Mooren's ulcer.[52] These peripheral corneal ulcers are associated with moderate infiltrate and vascularization and may be accompanied by scleritis. The peripheral corneal ulcers associated with Wegener's granulomatosis may respond to systemic immunosuppressives[53] and resections of the adjacent conjunctiva.

Scleritis is a well-recognized complication of rheumatoid arthritis. The scleritis can spread into and involve the adjacent cornea as a sclerokeratitis, and this may be associated with marginal thinning.[54] However, characteristic marginal corneal ulcers have been described in patients having rheumatoid arthritis without scleritis.[55] The characteristic marginal furrows of rheumatoid arthritis were observed in patients who had the disease for at least 5 years. The marginal furrows were located approximately 1 mm within the limbus and usually in the inferior cornea. The marginal thinning could be superficial and nonprogressive, or it could progress to epithelial breakdown, marked stromal thinning, and finally perforation. Usually there was minimal gross inflammation and vascularization, unless the lesion perforated. The marginal furrows may encircle the cornea, and bilateral involvement may be found. Occasionally, the entire superficial part of the remaining central island of corneal stroma may slough away. Topical corticosteroids must be used with extreme caution in patients having rheumatoid arthritis and associated peripheral corneal ulcers. Resection of the conjunctiva adjacent to these marginal ulcers may halt the ulcerative process.[56] The conjunctiva adjacent to peripheral corneal ulcers associated with rheumatoid arthritis has been shown to produce collagenase, and this may provide the basis for the beneficial effects of conjunctival resection.[57]

SUPERIOR LIMBIC KERATOCONJUNCTIVITIS (THEODORE)

Superior limbic keratoconjunctivitis (SLK), the syndrome first described and so named by Theodore in 1963,[58] has become a significant differential diagnostic consideration in external diseases, especially those conditions involving the upper cornea and/or corneal filaments. The disease is of unknown etiology and is characterized by a number of distinctive features: 1) marked inflammation of the tarsal conjunctiva of the upper lid; 2) inflammation of the upper bulbar conjunctiva; 3) fine punctate fluorescein or rose bengal staining of the cornea at the upper limbus and the adjacent conjunctiva above the limbus; 4) superior limbic proliferation and edema; and 5) in perhaps one-third of all attacks, the occurrence of filaments situated at the superior limbus or in the upper part of the cornea (Fig. 6.21). Although the filaments when present constitute the most outstanding feature of the entity, they are only a complication. The disease is much more common in females.[59, 60]

Cultures are essentially negative. Scrapings of the involved superior bulbar conjunctiva are valuable diagnostically, showing marked keratinization of the epithelial cells and polymorphs; scrapings of the palpebral conjunctiva reveal normal epithelium and a polymorphonuclear exudate. Biopsy specimens of the superior bulbar conjunctiva confirm findings on scrapings, showing prominent keratinization of the epithelium with acanthosis, dyskeratosis, cellular infiltration, and, in some areas, balloon degeneration of the nuclei.[61] Biopsy of the palpebral conjunctiva reveals infiltration with polymorphs, lymphocytes and plasma cells, and normal epithelium. Electron microscopic studies confirm the abnormal superior limbic epithelial changes.[62]

The frequent association of SLK with thyroid disease, originally noted by Tensel and others,[63–65] has suggested some immunological connection in which autoantibody reactions may be involved. However, our studies over some years have proved negative in regard to such an autoallergic or immune mechanism for the etiology of SLK. This opinion is supported by Eiferman and Wilkins,[66] who reported on three patients who had had therapeutic superior bulbar conjunctival resections for SLK. Clinical studies, biopsies, and other laboratory criteria of antibody dependence proved negative in all patients. Tests for thyroid dyscrasia were also negative in these patients.

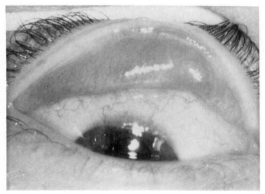

Figure 6.21 Theodore's superior limbic keratoconjunctivitis (SLK) characterized by upper tarsal conjunctivitis, superior bulbar injection, limbic proliferation and edema, superior corneal filaments (large ones at 2 o'clock). Diagnostic punctate staining of the involved bulbar conjunctiva and limbic cornea with fluorescein and rose bengal was also present.

DIAGNOSIS

SLK is generally readily recognized if the ophthalmologist is familiar with the entity, even if filaments are not present. Accurate diagnosis facilitates the best available therapy and the avoidance of harmful or ineffective measures. However, the following conditions may require differentiation: 1) trachoma, 2) superficial punctate keratitis (Thygeson), 3) marginal infiltrates (Fig. 6.22); 4) limbic

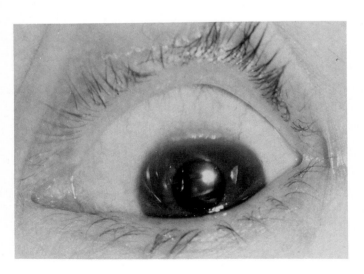

Figure 6.22 Marginal keratitis with injection of adjacent superior bulbar conjunctiva, apparently due to food allergy. Condition superficially resembled SLK, but neither tarsal conjunctivitis nor diagnostic staining with fluorescein and rose bengal were present. (Reprinted with permission from Theodore, F.H., and Schlossman, A. Ocular Allergy. Williams & Wilkins, Baltimore, 1958.)

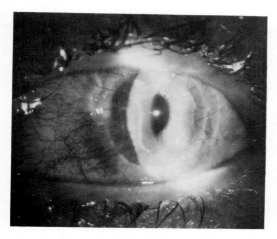

Figure 6.23 Epithelial rejection line after corneal transplantation.

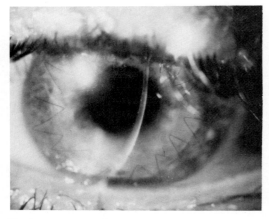

Figure 6.24 Early endothelial rejection showing inferior corneal edema.

lesions of vernal conjunctivitis, 5) phlyctenulosis, 6) other keratoconjunctivitis involving the upper palpebral conjunctiva, and 7) limbic tumors. In filamentary keratitis the upper corneal location of the filaments of SLK and its other distinctive features, especially its bulbar conjunctival staining, make its recognition not difficult.

TREATMENT

There is no specific treatment for SLK. Antibiotics, sulfonamides and corticosteroids are ineffectual. Generally, the most successful therapy is the topical application of ½% silver nitrate with a cotton applicator to the superior tarsal and superior bulbar conjunctiva on a weekly basis. This usually affords a marked relief of symptoms and the disappearance of filaments, if present, with eventual gradual improvement. Other methods include vasoconstrictors, acetylcysteine drops (not effective in our experience), cryotherapy, and surgical resection of the superior conjunctiva from 10 to 2 o'clock of an arcuate segment from the limbus to 5 mm above it.[67] Patching may prove valuable, especially, of course, where filaments have resulted in epithelial tears.[65] Soft lenses may also be of value in some cases of SLK[67a] particularly lenses of large size.[67b]

CORNEAL TRANSPLANTATION

Corneal transplantation enjoys a high success rate because the avascularity and absence of lymphatic drainage in this area bestow a considerable degree of immunological privilege. The absence of lymphatic vessels interferes with the afferent arc of the rejection process by reducing the chance of transplantation antigens coming into contact with patrolling lymphocytes.[68] The absence of blood vessels interferes with the efferent arc, preventing the entrance of rejecting cells to the transplanted tissue. It is more appropriate to say that the cornea enjoys an immunologically privileged site, rather than to say that the cornea is an immunologically privileged tissue, since the cornea itself possesses a reservoir of antigens in its cellular layers. Such antigens are referred to as "graft," "transplantation," or "histocompatibility" antigens since they are recognized and treated as foreign protein by lymphoid cells of the host. Khodadoust and Silverstein[69] have shown that all the cellular layers of the cornea may be involved in this rejection process.

Epithelial cell rejection can be seen as a fine line advancing across the cornea (Fig. 6.23). It consists of a necrotic zone of recipient epithelial cells infiltrated by inflammatory cells. Stromal rejection is manifested as an advancing layer of haziness caused by a pleomorphic cell population consisting of polymorphonuclear leukocytes, lymphocytes, and plasma cells. The manifestations of endothelial rejection include corneal edema, the appearance of mild anterior uveitis, and keratic precipitates on the posterior surface of the graft and an endothelial rejection line (Fig. 6.24). Subsequent destruction of the donor endothelium can result clinically in total corneal edema. The origin of the cells, in this type IV cell-mediated reaction, is thought to be either from the iris vessels (reaching the cornea through the aqueous) or from the limbal vessels (reaching the endothelium through an unhealed Descemet's membrane).[70] Allografts show an increased susceptibility to immunological rejection if there is pre-existing vascularization of the host. Once sensitization occurs, the vessels provide easy access to the graft. The majority of the corneal allografts survive irrespective of the degree of histocompatibility antigen correspondence because of the immunologically privileged site of the tissue. Where there has been previous sensitization or significant neovascularization, tissue typing may be of some practical advantage. The literature has not yet given a consistent answer as to the usefulness of HLA matching for high-risk cases of keratoplasty.[71]

The treatment of graft rejection requires topical corticosteroids, as well as periocular and oral corticosteroids when indicated. A suggested routine for severe rejection includes topical 1% prednisolone acetate or phostate hourly, triamcinolone acetonide 40 mg subconjunctivally weekly, and prednisone 60 mg orally each day for several days. Recently, cyclosporin A, an immunosuppressive with prominent inhibitory effects on T-lymphocytes, but minimal effects on B-lymphocytes, has been shown to suppress corneal allograft rejection in rabbits,[72] and may prove useful for corneal transplantation in humans as well.

REFERENCES

1. Theodore, F.H. Allergic keratitis. In Cornea World Congress, edited by King, Jr., J.H., and McTigue, J.W. Washington, Butterworths, 1965, pp. 197–206.
2. Theodore, F.H., Schlossman, A. Ocular Allergy. Williams & Wilkins, Baltimore, 1958.
3. Theodore, F.H. Idiosyncratic reactions of the cornea from proparacaine. Eye, Ear, Nose, Throat Monthly 47:296–291, 1968.
4. Duke-Elder, S. Diseases of the outer eye, Part 2, Cornea and sclera. In System of Ophthalmology, vol. 8. C.V. Mosby, St. Louis, 1965, pp. 815–839.
5. Cogan, D.G. Syndrome of nonsyphilitic interstitial keratitis and vestibuloauditory symptoms. Arch. Ophthalmol. 33:144, 1945.
6. Sorsby, A.P. The etiology of phlyctenular ophthalmia. Br. J. Ophthalmol. 26:159, 1942.
7. Thygeson, P. The etiology and treatment of phlyctenular keratoconjunctivitis. Am. J. Ophthalmol. 34:1217–1236, 1951.
8. Gibson, W.S. The etiology of phlyctenular conjunctivitis. Am. J. Dis. Child. 15:81–115, 1918.
9. Funaishi, S. Experimentelle Untersuchungen über die Aetiologie der phlyktänulären Augenentzündüngen. Klin. Monatsbl. Augenheilkd. 71:141–155, 1923.
10. Thygeson, P., Diaz-Bonnet, V., Okumoto, M. Phlyctenulosis: Attempts to produce an experimental model with BCG. Invest. Ophthalmol. 1:262–266, 1962.
11. Ballintine, E.J., Rotbart, D.C., Takimura, Y. Phlyctenulosis. Am. J. Ophthalmol. 73:459–460, 1972.
12. Mondino, B.J., Kowalski, R., Ratajczak, H.V., Peters, J., Cutler, S.B., Brown, S.I. Rabbit model of phlyctenulosis and catarrhal infiltrates. Arch. Ophthalmol. 99:891–895, 1981.
13. Thygeson, P. Complications of staphylococcic blepharitis. Am. J. Ophthalmol. 68:446, 1969.
14. Thygeson, P. Marginal corneal infiltrates and ulcers. Trans. Am. Acad. Ophthalmol. Otolaryngol. 51:198, 1947.
15. Smolin, G., Okumoto, M: Staphylococcal blepharitis. Arch. Ophthalmol. 95:812, 1977.
16. Mondino, B.J., Brown, S.I., Rabin, B.S.: The role of complement in corneal diseases. Trans. Ophthalmol. Soc. U.K. 98:363, 1978.
17. Cohn, H., Mondino, B.J., Brown, S.I., and Hall, G.D. Marginal corneal ulcers with beta streptococcal conjunctivitis and chronic dacryocystitis. Am. J. Ophthalmol. 87:541–543, 1979.
18. Buddingh, G.J., Schrum, D.I., Lanier, J.C., Guidry, D.J. Studies of the natural history of herpes simplex infection. Pediatrics 11:595, 1953.
19. Wander, A.H., Centifanto, Y.M., Kaufman, H.E. Strain specificity of clinical isolates of herpes simplex virus. Arch. Ophthalmol. 98:1458–1461, 1980.
20. Lopez, C., O'Reilly, R.J. Cell-mediated immune responses in recurrent herpes virus infections. J. Immunol. 118:875, 1977.
21. Lopez, C., Ryshke, R., Bloomfield, S. Adherent suppressor cells in patients with deep stromal disease associated with herpes keratitis. Invest. Ophthalmol. (ARVO Suppl) 17:273, 1978.
22. Metcalf, J.F., Kaufman, H.E.: Herpetic stromal

keratitis: Evidence for cell-mediated immuno-pathogenesis. Am. J. Ophthalmol. 82:527, 1976.

23. Lund, O.E., Stefani, F.H. Corneal histology after epidemic keratoconjunctivitis. Arch. Ophthalmol. 96:2085–2092, 1978.

24. Hogan, M.J. Atopic keratoconjunctivitis. Am. J. Ophthalmol. 36:937–947, 1953.

25. Rahi, A., Davies, P., Ruben, M., Lobascher, D., Menon, J. Keratoconus and coexisting atopic disease. Br. J. Ophthalmol. 61:761–764, 1977.

26. Brown, S.I., Shaninian, Jr., L. Diagnosis and treatment of ocular rosacea. Ophthalmology 85:779, 1978.

27. Jenkins, Mark S., Brown, S.I., Lempert, S.L., Weinberg, R.J. Ocular rosacea. Am. J. Ophthalmol. 88:618–622, 1979.

28. Dohlman, C.H., Boruchoff, S.A., Mobilia, E.F. Complications in use of soft contact lenses in corneal disease. Arch. Ophthalmol. 90:367–371, 1973.

29. Pitts, R.E., Krachmer, J.H. Evaluation of soft contact lens disinfection in the home environment. Arch. Ophthalmol. 97:470–472, 1979.

30. Gassett, A.R. Contact Lenses and Corneal Disease. Appleton-Century-Crofts, New York, 1979, pp. 254–257.

31. Smolin, G., Okumoto, M., Nozik, R. The microbial flora in extended-wear soft contact-lens wearers. Am. J. Ophthalmol. 88:543–547, 1979.

32. Mondino, B.J., Groden, L.R. Conjunctival hyperemia and corneal infiltrates with chemically disinfected soft contact lenses. Arch. Ophthalmol. 98:1767–1770, 1980.

33. Wilson, L.A., McNath, J., Reitschel, R. Delayed hypersensitivity to thimerosal in soft contact lens wearers. Ophthalmology 88:804–809, 1981.

34. Joondeph, H.C., McCarthy, W.L., Rabb, M., Constantaras, A.A. Mooren's ulcer: Two cases occurring after cataract extraction and treated with hydrophilic lens. Ann. Ophthalmol. 8:187, 1976.

35. Duke-Elder, S. Diseases of the outer eye. Part II. Cornea and sclera. In System of Ophthalmology, vol. 8. C.V. Mosby, St. Louis, 1965, pp. 914–920.

36. Linn, J.F. Chronic serpiginous ulcer of the cornea (Mooren's ulcer). Etiologic and therapeutic considerations. Am. J. Ophthalmol. 32:691, 1949.

37. Kuriakose, E.T. Mooren's ulcer. Etiology and treatment. Am. J. Ophthalmol. 55:1064, 1963.

38. Wood, T.O., Kaufman, H.E. Mooren's ulcer. Am. J. Ophthalmol. 71:417, 1971.

39. Brown, S.I. Mooren's ulcer. Histopathology and proteolytic enzymes of adjacent conjunctiva. Br. J. Ophthalmol. 59:670, 1975.

40. Feingold, M. Mooren's ulcer of the cornea. Am. J. Ophthalmol. 4:161, 1932.

41. Arentsen, J.J., Christiansen, J.M., Maumenee, A.E. Marginal ulceration after intracapsular cataract extraction. Am. J. Ophthalmol. 81:194, 1976.

42. Mondino, B.J., Brown, S.I., Mondzelewski, J.P. Peripheral corneal ulcers with herpes zoster ophthalmicus. Am. J. Ophthalmol. 86:611, 1978.

43. Aronson, S.B., Elliott, J.H., Moore, T.E., Jr., O'Day, D.M. Pathogenetic approach to therapy of peripheral corneal inflammatory disease. Am. J. Ophthalmol. 70:65, 1970.

44. Brown, S.I., Mondino, B.J., Rabin, B.S.: Autoimmune phenomenon in Mooren's ulcer. Am. J. Ophthalmol. 82:835, 1976.

45. Mondino, B.J., Brown, S.I., Rabin, B.S. Autoimmune phenomena of the external eye. Trans. Am. Acad. Ophthalmol. Otolaryngol. 85:801, 1978.

46. Eiferman, R.A., Hyndiuk, R.A. IgE in limbal conjunctiva in Mooren's ulcer. Canad. J. Ophthalmol. 12:234, 1977.

47. Mondino, B.J., Brown, S.I., Rabin, B.S.: Cellular immunity in Mooren's ulcer. Am. J. Ophthalmol. 85:788, 1978.

48. Brown, S.I. Mooren's ulcer. Treatment by conjunctival excision. Br. J. Ophthalmol. 59:675, 1975.

49. Maumenee, A.E. Lecture at University of California, San Francisco, 1972.

50. Brown, S.I., Mondino, B.J. Penetrating keratoplasty in Mooren's ulcer. Am. J. Ophthalmol. 89:255–258, 1980.

51. Wood, W.J., Nicholson, D.H. Corneal ring ulcer as the presenting manifestation of acute monocytic leukemia. Am. J. Ophthalmol. 76:69, 1973.

52. Cogan, D.G. Corneoscleral lesions in periarteritis nodosa and Wegener's granulomatosis. Trans. Am. Ophthalmol. 53:321, 1955.

53. Jampol, L.M., West, C., Goldberg, M.F. Therapy of scleritis with cytotoxic agents. Am. J. Ophthalmol. 86:266, 1978.

54. Jayson, M.I.V., Easty, D.L. Ulceration of the cornea in rheumatoid arthritis. Ann. Rheum. Dis. 36:428, 1977.

55. Brown, S.I., Grayson, M. Marginal furrows, a characteristic corneal lesion of rheumatoid arthritis. Arch. Ophthalmol. 79:563, 1968.

56. Wilson, F.M., Grayson, M., Ellis, F.D. Treatment of peripheral corneal ulcers by limbal conjunctivectomy. Br. J. Ophthalmol. 60:713, 1976.

57. Eiferman, R.A., Carothers, D.J., Yankeelow, J.A., Jr. Peripheral rheumatoid ulceration and evidence for conjunctival collagenase production. Am. J. Ophthalmol. 87:703, 1979.

58. Theodore, F.H. Superior limbic keratoconjunctivitis. Eye, Ear, Nose, Throat Monthly 42:25–28, 1963.

59. Theodore, F.H. Further observation on superior limbic keratoconjunctivitis. Trans. Am. Acad. Ophthalmol. Otolaryngol. 71:341–351, 1967.

60. Theodore, F.H. Superior limbic keratoconjunctivitis: Further studies. In Proceedings of the XXI International Congress of Ophthalmology. Excerpta Medica, Amsterdam, 1970, pp. 666–669.

61. Theodore, F.H., Ferry, A.P. Superior limbic keratoconjunctivitis—Clinical and pathological correlations. Arch. Ophthalmol. 84:481–484, 1970.

62. Donshik, P.E., et al. Conjunctival resection treatment and ultrastructural histopathology of superior limbic keratoconjunctivitis. Am. J. Ophthalmol. 85:101–110, 1978.

63. Tenzel, R.R. Comments on superior limbic keratoconjunctivitis. Arch. Ophthalmol. 79:508, 1968.

64. Cher, I. Clinical features of superior limbic keratoconjunctivitis in Australia: A probable association with thyrotoxicosis. Arch. Ophthalmol. 82:580–586, 1969.

65. Sutherland, A.L. Superior limbic keratoconjunctivitis: Report of a case. Trans. Ophthalmol. Soc. N.Z. 21:89–95, 1969.

66. Eiferman, R.A., Wilkins, E.L. Immunological aspects of superior limbic keratoconjunctivitis. Can. J. Ophthalmol. 14:85–87, 1979.

67. Tenzel, R.R. Resistant superior limbic keratoconjunctivitis. Arch. Ophthalmol. 89:439, 1973.

67a. Wright, P.: Superior limbic keratoconjunctivitis. Trans. Ophthalmol. Soc. U.K. 92:555–560, 1972.

67b. Mondino, B.J., Zaidman, G.W., Salamon, S.M.: Use of pressure patching and soft contact lenses in superior limbic keratoconjunctivitis. Arch. Ophthalmol. 100:1932–1934, 1982.

68. Billingham, R.E., Boswell, T. Studies on the problem of corneal homografts. Proc. R. Soc. Lond. [Biol] 141:392, 1953.

69. Khodadoust, A.A., Silverstein, A.M. Transplantation and rejection of individual cell layers of the cornea. Invest. Ophthalmol. 8:180, 1969.

70. Polack, F.M. Corneal graft rejection: Clinicopathological correlation. In Corneal Graft Failure. Ciba Foundation Symposium. Excerpta Medica, Amsterdam, 1973, p 127.

71. Stark, W.J., Taylor, H.R., Bias, W.B., Maumenee, A.E. HLA antigen and keratoplasty. Am. J. Ophthalmol. 86:595, 1978.

72. Salisbury, J.D., Gebhardt, B.M. Suppression of corneal allograft rejection by cyclosporin A. Arch. Ophthalmol. 99:1640–1643, 1981.

CHAPTER SEVEN

The Sclera and Episclera

The widespread use of anti-infective agents and the control of syphilis and tuberculosis have lessened the importance of infection in the causation of scleritis. Thus, while scleritis itself is a relatively infrequent disease, the percentage of scleral inflammations of probable immune origin is very high—perhaps higher than in any other ocular structure. However, because the sclera, unlike the conjunctiva, cornea, and uvea, does not lend itself so readily to the experimental investigation of allergic phenomena, it has been largely ignored in this respect. Until recently we have been forced to depend chiefly on clinical observations for the evaluation of the various immune mechanisms that appear to operate in the production of scleritis. The introduction of new laboratory tools to define immune mechanisms has given us more insight into the immunopathology of scleral disease.

Episcleritis is generally a benign recurrent disease, only rarely more serious than a nuisance to the patient.[1] It may be classified as nodular or simple (sectorial or diffuse). Scleritis not only can cause great pain and discomfort, but also may indicate serious systemic disease in half of those afflicted. In addition, if the patient develops necrotizing scleritis there is a one in five chance of dying in 8 years.[2] Anterior scleritis may be divided into diffuse, nodular or necrotizing, with and without adjacent inflammation. Posterior scleritis can also be found and should be suspected in unexplained cases of exudative retinal detachment, disc or macular edema and posterior uveitis. Topical vasoconstrictors may be useful in blanching the superficial episcleral plexus which is predominantly involved in episcleritis to reveal congestion of the deep episcleral plexus and underlying edema and necrosis of the sclera.

ATOPIC REACTIONS

Most atopic allergic reactions causing scleritis arise from foods, especially seafood and usually fish (Fig. 7.1). Inhalant allergies are rare but may occur from ragweed.

MICROBIALLERGIC REACTIONS

The sclera can be involved in systemic diseases of an infectious nature in which there is a direct invasion of the organism into the sclera with a granulomatous or hypersensitivity reaction to the organisms. Although rare today, the most likely endogenous infections involving the sclera are tuberculosis, leprosy, syphilis, and viral infection. It is important to identify this type of scleritis as being caused by an organism since the first three are amenable to specific therapy. If specific therapy is not used,, and treatment includes anti-inflammatory agents alone, the causative agents may proliferate through a depression of the host response and the disease may get worse.

There is some controversy over performing a scleral biopsy for diagnostic purposes. Scleral diseases have been known to get worse after biopsies. But it may be necessary to take a biopsy if a granulomatous process secondary to an organism is suspected. Epithelial scrapings, so useful in conjunctival and corneal disease, may be of use in this regard. Other systemic signs and laboratory studies may offer supporting evidence for a specific etiological agent.

Tuberculosis was once the most common cause of scleritis, either arising as an exogenous infection or in a generalized systemic miliary tuberculosis. Today, it is quite rare.

Histologically, in order to prove tuberculosis of the sclera, it is necessary to find not only granuloma formation, but also signs of the tubercle bacillus, such as a positive acid-fast stain or growth of the organisms on appropriate media (Fig. 7.2).

Scleral tuberculosis[3] represents a classic delayed hypersensitivity reaction or cell-mediated immune response to the tubercle bacillus, which may result in considerable inflammation but which may not be able to clear the host of the offending microorganism (Fig. 7.3).

In leprosy (Fig. 7.4) there are two clinically recognizable varieties of involvement, lepromatous and tuberculoid. In lepromatous leprosy, nodules are teeming with bacilli which the macrophage is unable to destroy. They appear on the iris, ciliary body, and sclera. Therefore, uveitis is frequently seen. If a lepromatous nodule arises close to the limbus, it has the appearance of a severe, limbal vernal conjunctivitis. The cornea can become involved by direct extension, producing an interstitial keratitis or a phlyctenular type of keratitis. Patients with this form of lep-

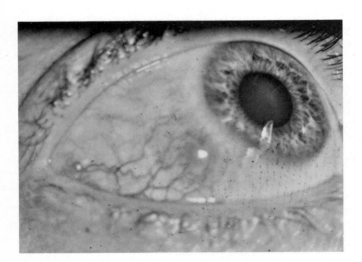

Figure 7.1 Nodular episcleritis apparently related to ingestion of various sea foods. (Reprinted with permission from Theodore, F.H. and Schlossman, A. Ocular Allergy. Williams & Wilkins, Baltimore, 1958.)

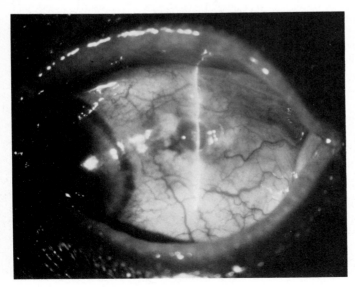

Figure 7.2 Active scleral tuberculosis.

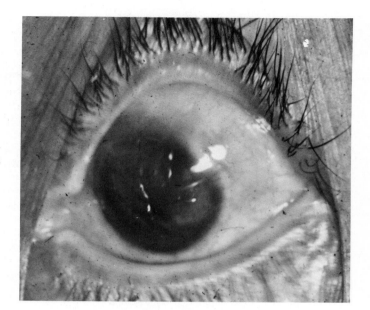

Figure 7.3 Sclerosing keratitis. Strongly positive tuberculin skin test.

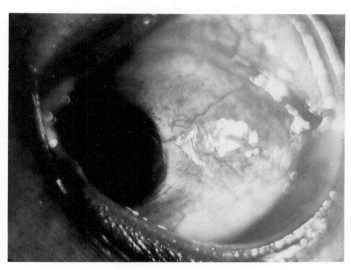

Figure 7.4 Scleritis in leprosy. (Courtesy of Dr. James H. Allen.)

rosy have impaired cellular immunity. The presence of large numbers of bacilli results in a marked humoral antibody response, and this in turn is associated with the formation of circulating immune complexes which are liable to provoke the type III hypersensitivity reaction in tissues.

In tuberculoid leprosy, cell-mediated immunological function is intact or possibly hyperactive. The tissue lesions are characterized by multiple granulomata and a paucity of demonstrable bacilli. A tendency for a granulomatous reaction to develop around peripheral nerves is the basis of most of the clinical manifestations of tuberculoid leprosy and is responsible for the lagophthalmos, exposure keratitis, and neurokeratitis.[4]

Syphilis, in Watson's experience, is a surprisingly common cause of scleritis. An investigation for syphilis should never be omitted when examining a patient with scleral disease. Not infrequently, scleritis is the presenting feature of the disease, and has been found associated with both anterior and posterior uveitis in two patients with necrotizing disease.[5]

Viral infections more commonly affect the conjunctiva and cornea than the sclera, but there are some important scleral involvements. Scleral and episcleral complications occur in 6% of patients with herpes zoster ophthalmicus.[5] The majority of patients with early episcleritis recover completely and have no residual changes; however, months to years later, 20% develop a severe necrotizing or nodular scleritis. This is often accompanied by a uveitis and a disciform keratitis which consists of deep stromal opacities, sometimes with immune rings which progress to a sclerosing keratitis. This type of necrotizing scleritis is extremely resistant to treatment.

SCLERITIS RELATED TO CONNECTIVE TISSUE DISORDERS

The central feature of the immune system is that it usually manages to distinguish quite precisely between normal body tissue and foreign material. In the so-called collagen diseases there is an apparent immunological reaction of the host against its own tissue. In autoimmune disease there exists the seemingly anomalous condition that Ehrlich referred to in 1900 as "horror autotoxicus," in which a self-destructive inflammatory process occurs directed by one's own immune system.[6]

Another way of looking at autoimmunity is to consider it as an immune reaction directed at an antigen whose inappropriate processing leads to inflammatory destruction of host tissues. This kind of inflammation is thought to occur in the scleritis seen with rheumatoid arthritis, polyarteritis nodosa, systemic lupus erythematosus, and Wegener's granulomatosis.

Postulated Immune Mechanism

There is increasing circumstantial evidence that immune complexes play an important role in the immunopathology of both systemic and eye involvement in these diseases.[7] Circulating immune complexes have a predilection for vascular basement membranes in target organs such as sclera, where they lodge, activate complement, initiate immunological inflammation, and ultimately cause tissue damage.

A major question involves the nature of the initiating factors. Is there an exogenous antigen, such as a virus, which triggers the reaction, or is there a factor which alters the cell surface characteristics of the patient's own cells, resulting in autoimmunity? In certain of the polyarteritis syndromes, hepatitis B virus has been found frequently.[8] It is postulated that this may be responsible for triggering the reaction. Another important consideration in understanding the pathophysiology of collagen disease is whether a genetic predisposition exists. The possibility that the genetic factor operates via immune mechanisms has received support from the observations that ankylosing spondylitis is associated with HLA-B 27. The clinical evidence for genetic influence in systemic lupus erythematosus (SLE) is supported by the SLE-like syndromes seen in patients with hereditary deficiencies of certain complement components.[9] The difficulty in detecting initiating factors may be because they are environmental agents which do not normally induce disease, but which in genetically susceptible individuals may do so by subtle interaction with the immune system. The next sections will consider individually some of those collagen diseases with scleral involvement.

Rheumatoid Arthritis

Rheumatoid arthritis is a classic example of an immune complex disease associated with scleritis. In this disease, an abnormal variant of the patient's IgG antibody becomes the antigen against which the patient develops rheumatoid factors (Rhf). These rheumatoid factors are predominantly IgM antibody. It is postulated that the union of rheumatoid factor antibodies with the antigenic IgG results in complement fixation and immunogenic inflammation.

In other words, we have a situation in which the patient's own IgG antibody or an abnormal variant of it becomes the antigen. The antigenic part of the IgG antibody has been shown to reside in the Fc portion of the heavy chain. Rheumatoid factor is thus characterized as an autoantibody or, more specifically, as an antiglobulin antibody. More recently, IgG, IgE, and IgA rheumatoid factors have been demonstrated. Therefore, the rheumatoid factors are antibodies of various classes which are directed against the Fc portion of the patient's own IgG antibodies.[10] The significance of rheumatoid factor is unclear. It forms the basis for the sheep agglutination and latex fixation test for rheumatoid arthritis.

In the central zone of scleral nodules in scleritis, Rhf appears to be directed against the patient's IgG which has become affixed to scleral collagen. It is postulated that union of the Rhf antibodies and the antigenic IgG results in complement fixation and immunogenic inflammation[11] (Fig. 7.5). The nodules often have an occluded vessel, suggesting that an occlusive vasculitis plays a role in the pathology. This may account for the scleral degeneration that follows nodule formation. The characteristic swelling of the necrotizing nodule is largely due to inflammatory edema and subsequent fibroblastic activity.

Joint synovium may act as an ectopic lymph node and produce or synthesize immunoglobulins. Such ability of the rheumatoid synovium to function as an ectopic lymph organ capable of intense local immunological activity is probably relevant to the role that it plays in perpetuating chronic inflammation which results in damage to the joint. In the joint

it is postulated that complexes of modified IgG and locally formed rheumatoid factors result in the activation of complement, thereby provoking the release of hydrolytic enzymes and subsequent erosions of the articular surfaces.[10] This sequence of events may also apply to the eye. The conjunctiva may function like the synovium in acting as an ectopic lymph node, causing disease of the underlying sclera.

There is nothing distinctive in the clinical appearance of the eye lesion that characterizes it as rheumatoid scleritis. The associated clinical history must be considered to determine whether or not this is a scleritis related to arthritis.

The most severe kind of disease is a necrotizing process, resulting in avascular areas with loss of scleral tissue either with or without inflammation. In certain patients, almost all of them female, with very severe longstanding arthritis and destructive joint changes, the scleral tissue almost completely disappears. This may take place without any obvious inflammatory change, which is then known as scleromalacia perforans. If there is a preceding extensive inflammatory condition, then the term necrotizing scleritis with inflammation is usually used, in which very discrete areas become necrotic with sequestrum formation.

Systemic Lupus Erythematosus (SLE)

SLE is another collagen disease in which scleral involvement is possible, although a retinal vasculitis is more com-

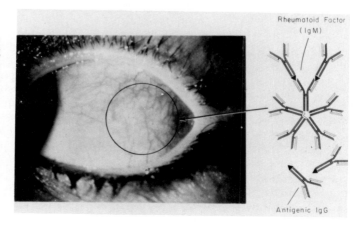

Figure 7.5 Composite diagram and photograph showing what is thought to be immune complex mediated rheumatoid scleritis. The patient's abnormal IgG antibody becomes the antigen. Rheumatoid factor (Rhf), mainly IgM, develops. Their union with the IgG and deposition with complement in scleral blood vessels results in what we clinically call scleritis.

Table 7.1
Clinical Reactions of the Sclera and Episclera

1. Atopic allergy (immediate reaction)
   a. Inhalants—episcleritis
   b. Food allergy—episcleritis
2. Microbial allergy may play a role
   a. *Streptococcus, Staphylococcus*—episcleritis, scleritis
   b. Tubercle and lepra bacilli—scleritis, sclerosing keratitis
   c. Other microorganisms—episcleritis, scleritis
   d. Herpes zoster—scleritis, sclerokeratitis
3. Collagen diseases (immune complex-mediated disease)
   a. Rheumatoid arthritis, polyarteritis, lupus erythematosus—scleritis, necrotizing scleritis

mon. In rheumatoid arthritis there are autoantibodies, rheumatoid factors (Rhf), directed against an abnormal immunoglobulin G molecule. In lupus, there are autoantibodies directed against antigenic constitutents in the nucleus and cytoplasm of patients' leukocytes. The leukocyte nucleus undergoes denaturation and phagocytosis because of an antibody directed against a component of the nucleus. The first antinuclear factor discovered was directed against deoxyribonucleoprotein. It is responsible for the lupus erythematosus (LE) cell phenomenon. Antinuclear factors have also been found against other chemical components of the leukocyte nucleus. The LE cell factor is an IgG antibody. It is also called antinuclear antibody or ANA. The LE cell is a polymorphonuclear leukocyte that has ingested nuclear material complexed with antinuclear antibody. Therefore, it appears that in SLE, autoimmune phenomenona develop against nuclear and cytoplasmic constituents of host cells. How the autoimmune phenomenona develop is the key question.[12]

Associated with both rheumatoid arthritis and SLE is a triad consisting of keratoconjunctivitis sicca, xerostomia, and the connective tissue disorder. The combination of xerophthalmia and xerostomia alone is often referred to as the sicca syndrome. Biopsy of the affected lacrimal

and salivary glands shows heavy infiltration of the tissue with mononuclear cells, both lymphocytes and plasma cells. Patients with Sjögren's syndrome show an apparently increased tendency to develop lymphoreticular malignancy and pseudolymphoma.[13]

Vasculitis

The term "vasculitis" is used to describe conditions in which vessel walls show evidence of damage initiated by an inflammatory process. In practice, a diagnosis of vasculitis is often made on the basis of well-recognized clinical syndromes, with the aid of microscopic tissues where practical. Clinically, a majority of patients show no known initiating agents, although typical lesions of vasculitis have occurred in conjunction with infections or exposure to drugs. The unifying concept in the vascular diseases is that immune complexes mediate vascular damage. A vasculitis stage is seen in rheumatoid arthritis and SLE. Usually this occurs in an advanced and accelerated stage of the disease. In the vasculitis syndromes, granulomas or frankly destructive lesions may occur. All of these conditions are characterized by inflammation of blood vessels. There appears to be a spectrum of disease ranging from polyarteritis at one end (in which there is little or no granulomatous change but considerable change in the arteries) to Wegener's granulomatosis in which there is a substantial granulomatous reaction but relatively little vasculitis.

In polyarteritis nodosa, a necrotizing scleritis can occur which is quite severe (Fig. 7.6). There is an antigen-antibody reaction with complement fixation which takes place in the blood vessels of the sclera. The immune complex is then digested by polymorphonuclear leucocytes attracted to the site of deposition, and more inflammation results. Because of the characteristic pattern of deposition, immunofluorescent microscopy is often helpful in making the diagnosis of immune complex disease[14] (Fig. 7.7). The antigen in polyarteritis is unknown, but hepatitis B virus has been found in a high association, as noted earlier.

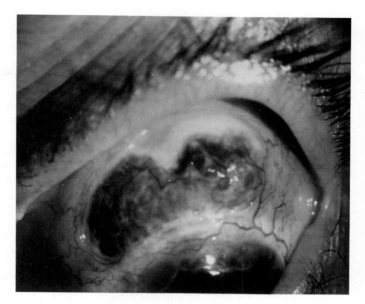

Figure 7.6 Necrotizing scleritis in polyarteritis nodosa.

IMMUNE COMPLEX DISEASE

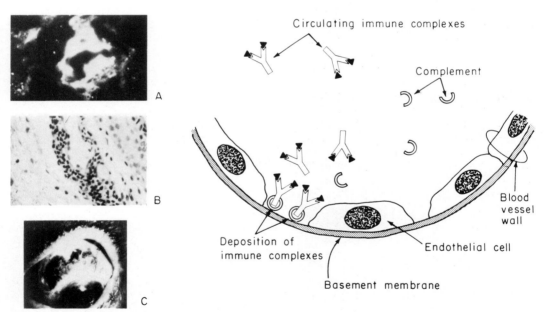

Figure 7.7 Necrotizing scleritis in polyarteritis—immune complex disease. Freely circulating immune complexes seem to have a predilection for basement membranes that underlie endothelial cells of blood vessels. Immunopathologically, immune complex disease is characterized by deposition of antigen-antibody and subsequent complement fixation on these basement membranes. *A*, immunofluorescent studies are helpful in making the diagnosis of immune complex disease. They have a characteristic granular (lumpy-bumpy) appearance. *B*, immune complexes are then digested by polymorphonuclear leukocytes attracted to the site of deposition. This results in more inflammation. Histology shows vessel infiltrated with inflammatory cells. *C*, clinically, one sees tissue destruction due to immune complex deposition, as in this case of necrotizing scleritis.

TREATMENT

The treatment of scleritis, at various stages, is controversial. There are many anti-inflammatory agents available, but only a few are effective in the treatment of scleral disease. These include systemic corticosteroids, indomethacin, oxyphenylbutazone, and, in some cases, antimitotic agents. Topical steroids are often, but not always, effective in episcleritis and, sometimes, in more superficial forms of scleritis. Systemic steroids are more effective. Often large doses are required, which should be used with caution especially in necrotizing scleritis. Subconjunctival injections of steroids appear to be especially inadvisable since they may result in extreme scleral thinning and, sometimes, perforation.[5]

GOUT

Gout,[15] an essentially metabolic disease, may be associated with both episcleritis and scleritis (Fig. 7.8). In fact, routine serum uric acid studies in scleritis often reveal unsuspected gout. An allergic component may contribute to the acute episodes of the disease.

TENONITIS

Except for the rare instance of tenonitis arising from direct infection, such as that complicating trauma or extraocular muscle surgery, the obscure origin of tenonitis appears best explained in certain instances on the basis of allergy. The rarity of the disease makes etiological evaluation difficult. Its exudative character with extreme chemosis (Fig. 7.9); its transient, recurrent, yet benign, course; its association with collagen disease; its relationship and similarity to scleritis; its response to corticosteroids and foreign protein therapy—all these characteristics suggest that an allergic component may play a role in its causation. However, we know of no known instance in which tenonitis has arisen on the basis of atopy, such as food allergy. In this regard it is possible that the chemosis and other ocular findings in trichinosis are due to tenonitis arising secondary to muscle infestation, either as a

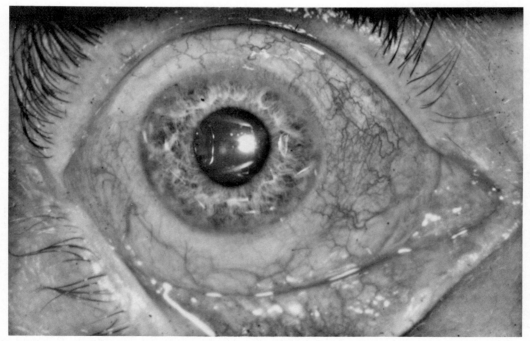

Figure 7.8 Episcleritis in gout. (Reprinted with permission from Theodore, F.H. and Schlossman, A. Ocular Allergy. Williams & Wilkins, Baltimore, 1958.)

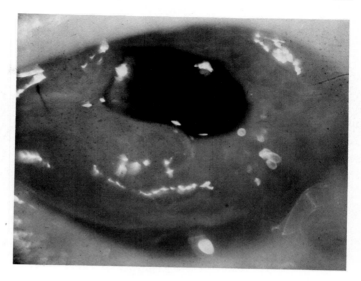

Figure 7.9 Severe serous sclerotenonitis showing marked chemosis, which differentiates condition from orbital cellulitis. (Reprinted with permission from Theodore, F.H. and Schlossman, A. Ocular Allergy. Williams & Wilkins, Baltimore, 1958.)

toxic or allergic response to products of the *Trichinella*.

Sclerotenonitis may be associated with rheumatoid arthritis. It may be associated with muscle paresis, usually involving the inferior and lateral recti, with diplopia. This responds dramatically to systemic steroids.

EXPERIMENTAL MODEL OF SCLERITIS

Rabbits were sensitized over a prolonged period to ovalbumin mixed with complete Freund's adjuvant by intradermal injection.[16] After injection of ovalbumin into the limbus, corneoscleral lesions developed that resembled necrotizing scleritis in humans. These lesions were destructive and progressive and typically showed a diffuse granulomatous reaction of the sclera and adjacent cornea with many plasma cells and lymphocytes. It was not determined whether the humoral response to ovalbumin alone or in combination with a cell-mediated response to some tissue antigen was responsible for the scleral lesions.

REFERENCES

1. Watson, P.G., Hayreh, S.S. Scleritis and episcleritis. Br. J. Ophthalmol. 60:163–191, 1976.
2. McGavin, D.D.M., Williamson, J., Forrester, J.V., Foulds, W.S., Buchanan, W.W., Dick, W.C., Lee, P., MacSween, R.N.M., Whaley, K. Episcleritis and scleritis. Br. J. Ophthalmol. 60:192–226, 1976.
3. Bloomfield, S.E., Mondino, B., Gray, G.P. Scleral tuberculosis. Arch. Ophthalmol. 94:954, 1976.
4. Friedlaender, M.H. Allergy and Immunology of the Eye. Harper and Row, Hagerstown, 1979, pp. 143–144.
5. Watson, P.G., Hazleman, B.L. The Sclera and Systemic Disorders. W.B. Saunders, London, 1976.
6. Bellanti, J.A. Immunologically mediated diseases. In Immunology, 11 ed., edited by Bellanti, J.A. W.B. Saunders, Philadelphia, 1978, p. 565.
7. Cooke, T.D., Hurd, E.R., Ziff, M., Hugo, E.J. The pathogenesis of chronic inflammation in experimental antigen-induced arthritis. II. Preferential localization of antigen antibody complexes to collagenous tissues. J. Exp. Med. 135:323–338, 1972.
8. Gocke, D., Hsu, J., Morgan, C., Lockshin, M., Bombardieri, S., Christian, C.L. Association between polyarteritis and Australia antigen. Lancet II:1149–1153, 1970.
9. Lachmann, F. Genetics of the complement system. J. Med. Genet. 12:372, 1975.
10. Maini, R.N., Glass, D.N., Scott, J.T. Immunology of the Rheumatic Diseases, Aspects of Autoimmunity. Edward Arnold, London, 1977, pp. 53–70.
11. Nowoslawski, A., Brzosko, W.J. Immunopathology of rheumatoid arthritis. II. The rheumatoid nodule. Pathol. Eur. 2:302–321, 1967.
12. Maini, R.N., Glass, D.N., Scott, J.T. Immunology of the Rheumatic Diseases, Aspects of Autoimmunity. Edward Arnold, London, 1977, pp. 71–88.
13. Maini, R.N., Glass, D.N., Scott, J.T. Immunology of the Rheumatic Diseases, Aspects of Autoimmunity. Edward Arnold, London, 1977, p. 92.

14. Bloomfield, S.E., Becker, C.G., Christian, C.L., Nauheim, J.S. Bilateral necrotizing scleritis with marginal corneal ulceration after cataract surgery in patient with vasculitis. Br. J. Ophthalmol. 64:170, 1980.

15. Theodore, F.H., Schlossman, A. Ocular Allergy. Williams & Wilkins, Baltimore, 1958, p. 315.

16. Hembry, R.M., Playfair, J., Watson, P.G., Dingle, J.T. Experimental model for scleritis. Arch. Ophthalmol. 97:1337–1340, 1979.

CHAPTER EIGHT

The Uvea

Anatomically, the extremely vascular uvea offers a favorable site for the interplay of various components of immune reactions. The major actor in the immune response, the lymphocyte, is not native to the eye but is attracted to it by the presence of antigen. The processing of antigen also does not take place in the eye, but at a distant site with a subsequent migration of sensitized lymphocytes towards an antigenic source in the eye. Once there, the immune factories or lymphocytes engage in humoral antibody formation, or cell-mediated reactions, depending upon the type of antigenic stimulation. It has been postulated by some authors that after the primary ocular response to antigenic challenge is over, a few lymphocytes or memory cells may persist in the uveal tissue, since a subsequent exposure to the same antigen introduced at a distant site or injected directly into the circulation results in renewed antibody production in the eye.[1]

In other words, the uveal tract may be acting as a regional lymph node, with subsequent exposure to antigen-stimulating memory cells to produce an immune reaction. This suggests that some cases of recurrent uveitis may be comparable to a lymphadenopathy, and the inflammation is really a physiological response to a prior antigenic stimulation. Unfortunately, a secondary or anamnestic response of this kind which might pass unnoticed in peripheral lymph nodes gives rise to clinically evident disease in the eye. Since the eye is a closed system, any signs of inflammatory or immune response will be manifested in symptomatology and clinically evident problems.

Since the uvea thus affords such an ideal shock organ for the study of allergic reactions, it is not surprising that investigators in the field of immunology have utilized this structure experimentally in the production of allergic reactions ever since the introduction of the concept of anaphylaxis. A great deal of the basic knowledge concerning hypersensitivity stems from such experiments. Allergic uveitis has been induced in laboratory animals by means of horse, cat, and other foreign sera, egg albumin, various microbial products, and by tissue proteins, either alone or in combination with complete Freund's adjuvant (heat-killed tubercle bacilli in mineral oil).

The foregoing observations reveal that all forms of allergic mechanisms operate in the production of uveal inflammation. Work by Silverstein and Zimmerman[2] confirms this by indicating that endophthalmitis may be produced in the guinea pig by two distinct immunological mechanisms: 1) delayed hypersensitivity; and 2) antigen interaction with circulating antibody. By varying the method of sensitization, the route of administration, and the dose of antigen, the several immunological mechanisms may be stimulated to produce ocular lesions.

The classification in Table 8.1 is useful for the understanding of the clinical manifestations of uveal hypersensitivity. It is an attempt to approach the problem of uveitis with a mechanistic method based upon the immune reaction involved. Hypersensitivity or allergic reactions of the immune response may occur and result in disease. On the other hand, deficiency in the immune response may result in a low resistance to infection and the emergence of infections by organisms previously considered benign, i.e., immunodeficiency or opportunistic uveitis.

Table 8.1
Clinical Reactions of the Uvea
_____

1. Atopic or anaphylactic uveitis—serum, food, drugs, proteins, angioneurotic edema
2. Microbiallergic uveitis
   a. Bacterial—_Streptococcus_, tuberculosis, syphilis
   b. Viral—herpes simplex, varicella-zoster
   c. Fungal—histoplasmosis
   d. Protozoan—Toxoplasmosis
   e. Helminthic—onchocerciasis, _Toxocara_
3. Autoimmune uveitis
   a. Phacoanaphylaxis (lens-induced uveitis)
   b. Sympathetic ophthalmia
   c. Vogt-Koyanagi-Harada syndrome (?)
4. Uveitis of possible immune origin
   a. Recurrent endogenous iritis—immune complex disease with increased vascular permeability (?)
   b. Behcet's disease—immune complex disease
   c. Sarcoidosis—cell-mediated immunity
5. Immunodeficiency uveitis (opportunistic uveitis)
   a. Metastatic endophthalmitis with non-pathogenic organisms
   b. Role of stress in triggering uveitis in immunocompetent patients
_____

HYPERSENSITIVITY REACTIONS

Hypersensitivity reactions, manifested as a uveitis, may represent hypersensitivity to either exogenous antigens or autologous tissue components. The exogenous antigens may be of an infectious or non-infectious nature. Given the present state of the art, we are unlikely to know what the inciting antigen is.

ATOPIC OR ANAPHYLACTIC UVEITIS

Anaphylactic and atopic reactions of the uvea, though rare, offer the best clinical corroboration of the fact that the uvea may be involved in generalized allergic reactions.

This type of reaction is probably rare because of the reduced opportunity for direct contact of the antigen with the uvea, in contrast to such tissues as the conjunctiva, where contact is readily achieved and an allergic response relatively frequent. There are many scattered case reports of alleged examples of uveal tract involvement caused by so-called allergies. Instances of atopic allergic uveitis are said to have occurred from hypersensitivity to ragweed, house dust, cat dander, and other inhalants and to foods. But such reports must be viewed critically, awaiting confirmation through more refined diagnostic techniques which show that these reactions are definitely IgE mediated. In 1973, Bloch-Michel[3] suggested strict criteria for the diagnosis of atopic or anaphylactic uveitis. He argued that there must be collateral evidence of hypersensitivity affecting other tissues of family members, a positive skin test, a provocation of uveal signs by administration of a test dose of the suspected allergen, and remission of allergy in response to specific desensitization. These criteria appear somewhat strict because, for one thing, remission of allergy after desensitization is by no means an automatic sequel to such therapy.

Serum reactions offer the best evidence, both clinically and experimentally, that allergic uveitis is a definite entity. Serum sickness is a systemic disease caused by injection of a foreign serum such as horse serum antitoxin. The injected protein serves as an immediate immunogen, then persists in tissue long enough to act as an eliciting antigen for a type III reaction. Therefore, the acute manifestations of serum sickness are due to IgE-mediated (type I) damage, and the chronic symptoms are associated with immune complex deposition.[4] The uveitis associated with serum sickness was originally described by Theodore and Lewson in 1939[5] and has been produced experimentally by many investigators. An even more remarkable instance of bilateral iridocyclitis due to foreign serum was reported by Sedan and Guillot in 1955.[6] The patient received tetanus antitoxin on three different occasions over a period of 6 years. Each time bilateral iridocyclitis occurred with a lessened interval between injection and the onset of symptoms, a true anamnestic reaction. Papillitis, with retinal edema and hemorrhages, has also been noted in serum sickness.

MICROBIALLERGIC UVEITIS

The primary uveal response to pyogenic bacteria is an acute inflammatory reaction with an initial outpouring of polymorphonuclear leukocytes. Immunological activity is manifested after a latent period of several days and is essentially protective in character. Failure of the cellular and humoral mechanisms to eradicate the offending organism can lead to chronic infection and the development of immunological hypersensitivity. A division into nongranulomatous and granulomatous inflammation on the assumption that granulomatous formation represents the presence of living organisms is not completely valid. Actually, granuloma formation can be provoked by immune complexes, and organismal infection may evoke a nongranulomatous reaction. In general, however, patients with uveitis secondary to an organism call forth a cell-mediated immune response often resulting in granuloma formation.

A partial list of bacterial organisms considered over the years to cause uveitis includes the infectious agents of tuberculosis, syphilis, brucellosis, and streptococcus, gonococcus, and pneumococcus. The real incidence and role of these organisms in causing uveitis is unclear and has probably been overstated in the past.

Viruses also cause uveitis. The two most common are herpes simplex and varicella-zoster virus. It is unclear whether herpes simplex uveitis is due to direct viral infection of the uveal tract or whether hypersensitivity mechanisms are responsible.[7] In addition, some immunosuppression of the host may play a role in the initiation of these infections (see later section on opportunistic uveitis).

There are a number of pathogenic fungi that result in disease in people with an intact immunological defense system. Histoplasmosis is a fungus endemic to certain areas of the world. It is also postulated that the presumed ocular histoplasmosis syndrome (Fig. 8.1), so named because the organism is seldom isolated, may be occasionally produced by agents other than *Histoplasma capsulatum*. The granuloma formation and pulmonary tissue destruction seen in histoplasmosis are generally attributed to vigorous cell-mediated immune responses to the infection.[8] On the other hand, cell-mediated immunity may fail in disseminated histoplasmosis. Humoral immune responses also develop in

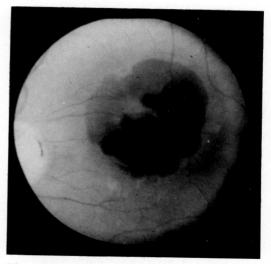

Figure 8.1 Ocular histoplasmosis. (Courtesy of Dr. Robert S. Coles.)

histoplasmosis. Antibodies are not protective, but rather indicate progressive disease. The flareup of macular disease following a skin test with histoplasmin may be due to the heightened cellular immune mechanisms.[9]

Protozoal uveitis can be caused by *Toxoplasma gondii*, an obligatory intracellular parasite. It is thought to account for 25% of all uveitis cases in Britain. It most commonly results in a focal necrotizing retinitis (discussed in Chapter 9).

Helminthic uveitis may be caused by *Onchocerca volvulus* and *Toxocara canis*. Live microfilaria of the Onchocerca cause little or no reaction. Tissue response to onchocerciasis is promoted by dead organisms. It is not clear to what extent the inflammatory reaction can be ascribed to direct toxicity of products of the dying organism or to immunological responses with a strongly allergic component. Moreover, in common with other helminthic infestations, serum levels of IgE are elevated and eosinophils form a prominent component of the cellular exudates in sectioned tissues. *Toxocara* is primarily a retinal manifestation (discussed under that heading). The role of steroids in the treatment of these diseases presents a problem. Steroids dampen the harmful inflammatory ocular response, but they also depress the immune defense mechanisms responsible for clearing the organism.

AUTOIMMUNE UVEITIS

Long before the concept of autoallergy or sensitization of the host to his own tissues was utilized to explain certain systemic diseases, the ophthalmologist recognized that two unique types of autogenous allergy occur in the eye, phacoanaphylactic uveitis and sympathetic ophthalmia.

Phacoanaphylaxis

In 1899 Schirmer[10] wrote that the toxic properties of lens material were responsible for the delayed and severe irritant properties of lens protein following extracapsular cataract extraction. The possibility that immune factors may play a role was first suggested by Verhoeff and Lemoine in 1922.[11]

The lens is immunologically isolated by virtue of its anatomic position in an avascular aqueous medium and the possession of a capsule lined with epithelium, normally preventing both egress of potential antigens and entry of antibodies and immune competent cells. Each of the crystalline protein groups in the lens contains distinct antigenic characteristics. Even so, autologous lens proteins are only weakly antigenic and even when liberated into the aqueous, frequently fail to elicit an immune response. Clinically, phacoanaphylactic endophthalmitis appears to be a definite hypersensitivity reaction, but because its experimental production in animals has required adjuvants in addition to the lens protein, some investigators believe that there are other factors required to trigger the immune mechanism. Some adjuvant combining with lens protein is possibly operative in this case.

However, clinical experience with the use of fish lens extract in the treatment of cataract in humans offers excellent experimental confirmation of 1) the allergic basis for endophthalmitis phacoanaphylactica, and 2) the organ specificity, rather than species specificity, of allergy to lens protein. Uveitis has been induced by repeated injections of fish lens protein and cured by intracapsular cataract extraction.[12,13] Some people prefer the terms phacoantigenic uveitis or lens-induced uveitis rather than the more historical term, phacoanaphylactic endophthalmitis.

Characteristically, lens-induced uveitis develops 1–14 days after traumatic or surgical perforation of the lens capsule with liberation of lens material. Clinically it may be extremely severe, with lid and corneal edema, mutton-fat keratic precipitates, posterior synechiae, and formation of a cyclitic membrane. Uveitis affects the iris principally, the choroid only secondarily. The demonstration that lens trauma in previously sensitized animals leads to the in vivo fixation of IgG and complement lends support to the suggestion that lens-induced endophthalmitis is an immune complex disease.[14] It is believed that lens proteins are tolerated rather than totally sequestered and that autoimmune disease results only when T-cell tolerance is altered or bypassed.[14a] Occasionally a patient who has had a lens-induced inflammation in one eye may develop a similar or more pronounced uveal reaction in the second eye at a later date. This type of response appears to depend on the lens in the second eye being cataractous or suffering a traumatic rupture, thus exposing the sequestered antigens of the lens protein. It is probable that the response in the second eye is due to an anamnestic response or a restimulation of already primed lymphoid tissue. Occasionally bilateral lens-induced reactions can be confused with sympathetic ophthalmia.[15] An acute lens-induced uveitis with secondary glaucoma may also occur spontaneously in patients with hypermature cataracts.

Sympathetic Ophthalmia

Analysis of experimental and clinical knowledge concerning sympathetic ophthalmia (SO) indicates that the most acceptable pathogenesis of this entity is some form of hypersensitivity. The immune reaction apparently required special exciting factors, some of which are still unknown.

The immunological aspects of SO have been more widely studied than those of almost any other ocular disease. Yet it has not been easy to establish the immunopathogenesis of SO, and it remains unclear what antigen and which effector mechanisms are important in this disease.

Historically, Elschnig in 1910[16] proposed that uveal pigment was the offending antigen. Woods[17] expanded the concept and demonstrated that patients with SO had cellular reactivity to a crude extract of uveal antigen.

Friedenwald,[18] utilizing histological skin studies of people who received such intradermal injections of suspensions of uveal pigment, believed that the uveal pigment granules acted as a specific antigen and that the disease was primarily allergic in nature.

Other investigators suggest that the allergic reaction resulting in sympathetic ophthalmia is somewhat more complicated and requires special circumstances for its development. Collins[19] working with guinea pigs, found it was necessary to employ complete Freund's adjuvant in addition to uveal pigment to produce the reaction. Naquin,[20] however, was unable to duplicate this work. Blodi[15] analyzed 170 eyes with SO and found that 39, or about 23%, showed evidence of a phacoanaphylactic reaction. He believed that this association was higher than could be expected by chance coincidence and that the simultaneous occurrence lent additional weight to the concept of an allergic pathogenesis in sympathetic uveitis.

Recent studies have concentrated on the possible role of cellular immunity in the pathogenesis of SO. This is suggested by the virtual absence of plasma cells in the cellular infiltrate, the absence of a significant antibody response, the demonstration that experimental allergic uveitis in guinea pigs can be passively transferred by the injection of lymphocytes but not by serum,[21] and the finding by Marak and co-workers in 1973 of T-lymphocyte sensitization in some cases of uncomplicated perforated eye injuries but not in endogenous uveitis. The evidence for autosensitization to uveal antigens is strong, but there is no good evidence that the reaction is damaging to the uveal tissues. There is no doubt that autoimmune phenomena can and do occur in the uvea; the real problem concerns the relevance of the phenomena to the initiation and maintenance of uveitis. Antigens specific for the uvea are generally considered to be associated with the pigment-containing cells. In general, tissue specific antigens tend to be located inside cells and do not make ready contact with patrolling lymphocytes. They may therefore be regarded as sequestered antigens which will evoke an immune response only if released by tissue destruction. The overall antigenicity of uveal proteins is low and antibody responses in animals given homologous extracts rapidly disappear when the stimulus is withdrawn. Moreover, there is frequently no effect at all unless the extracts are combined with Freund's adjuvant, and even then a detectable response may be lacking. In addition, there is some question as to whether uveal pigment is the inciting agent. Some investigators consider that retinal pigment epithelium and photoreceptor outer limbs provide the more effective stimuli to homologous uveitis than the uvea itself.[23]

Wacker[24] and co-workers have demonstrated and partially characterized the antigen in the photoreceptor and retinal pigment epithelial layers that can elicit the development of chorioretinitis. They refer to the inciting agent as the S-antigen (soluble), which has been located throughout the photoreceptor layer.

The beneficial effects of immunosuppressive drug therapy also suggest that SO is an autoimmune disease. In summary, there is strong, but not conclusive evidence that SO results from autoimmune phenomena mediated mainly by the T-lymphocyte through the cell-mediated immune response. There is some question concerning the most important antigenic stimulant. The overall antigenicity of uveal proteins is low. That is why some investigators have postulated that retinal pigment epithelium and photoreceptor outer limbs may be the effective stimulus resulting in the uveitis.

Posterior Uveitis

It is believed that the S-antigen experimental autoimmune uveitis model may be the model most relevant to human disease because patients with posterior uveitis show cell-mediated immunity to this antigen and because there are similar clinicopathological features in humans and in the animal model.[24a] Experimental autoimmune uveitis may be inhibited by cyclosporin A, demonstrating that T-cells participate in this disease. Interestingly, patients with birdshot retinochoroidopathy also show positive cellular immunity to purified retinal S-antigen, which may play a role in this disease.[24b]

Vogt-Koyanagi-Harada Syndrome

Vogt-Koyanagi-Harada (VKH) syndrome appears histopathologically similar to SO. They both result in a granulomatous uveitis. A common origin for both diseases has long been suspected. There is a heightened cellular and humoral reactivity to uveal antigen but its significance is unclear.[25]

UVEITIS OF POSSIBLE IMMUNE ORIGIN

The cause of recurrent endogenous iritis remains a mystery, but a model for recurrent iritis has been developed. It involves the concepts of immune complex disease and increased vascular permeability. It is postulated that a severe primary nonimmune inflammation of the uveal tract, regardless of etiology, may result in a prolonged increase in vascular permeability of the uveal vessels. A subsequent antigen-antibody reaction could then result in deposition of immune complexes in tissue altered by previous inflammation. Subsequent antigen-antibody complexes may be etiologically unrelated to the primary insult. So, any time the body is reacting to inflammation with an antigen-antibody reaction, a recurrent iritis would occur because of increased vascular permeability caused by prior damage to uveal vessels. This tendency of vessels injured by nonimmune damage in one part of the body to become more permeable with subsequent immune (antigen-antibody) reactions in other parts of the body has been called the Auer reaction, after its discoverer. It remains to be seen if this attractive hypothesis is indeed the cause of recurrent iritis.

Behcet's Syndrome

Behcet was a Turkish dermatologist, who, in 1937,[26] described a triad of signs consisting of recurrent iritis and recurrent oral and genital ulcerations. The oral ulceration is so constant that it forms the cornerstone of the diagnosis. These painful oral lesions consist of variously sized and shaped aphthous ulcers in different parts of the mouth[27] (Fig. 8.2). Genital ulcers also tend to be recurrent and are mainly single in the male but multiple in the female.

Ocular lesions are common, occurring in approximately 75% of patients with Behcet's syndrome. The most common presenting sign is an iridocyclitis with a hypopyon (Fig. 8.3), which may resolve with or without treatment. Other ocular manifestations include choroiditis, retinal phlebitis, and arteritis. Ocular complications include cataract formation and glaucoma from the recurrent iritis.

The immunopathology of Behcet's syndrome appears to be a vasculitis with early infiltration of vessels by mononuclear cells, and later infiltration by polymorphonuclear cells. Lehner[28] believes that immune complexes of the IgA, IgG,

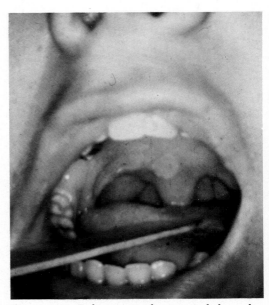

Figure 8.2 Behcet's syndrome. Aphthous lesions of the soft palate.[27] (Courtesy of Dr. Helen O. Curth.)

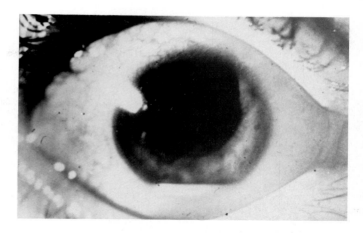

Figure 8.3 Behcet's syndrome. Iritis with hypopyon. This eye had been operated on for secondary glaucoma, because of uveitis.[27] (Courtesy of Dr. Helen O. Curth.)

and IgM classes play an essential part in the pathogenesis of Behcet's syndrome. Significant elevation of immune complexes has been found in the serum of patients with this disease.[29] Corticosteroids and chlorambucil have been used to treat the manifestations of this syndrome.

Sarcoidosis

Sarcoidosis is a systemic disease characterized by the infiltration of affected tissue by noncaseating tuberculoid granulomata. Approximately one-fourth of patients with sarcoidosis have ocular manifestations which can involve virtually any tissue of the eye.

Uveitis is the most frequent ocular complication[30] and can present as an acute iridocyclitis, a chronic iridocyclitis with multiple discrete granulomata on the iris (Fig. 8.4), or a posterior uveitis characterized by "candle wax drippings." Sarcoidosis is the usual cause of Heerfordt's syndrome, in which generalized uveitis is accompanied by painless swelling of the parotid glands, fever, lymph node enlargement, splenomegaly, and polyneuritis. Lid, conjunctival, lacrimal gland, and orbital involvement have all been reported.

There are characteristic alterations in the cell-mediated immune response, but it is unclear whether they represent a primary immunological disturbance or whether the abnormalities are secondary to widespread inflammation of lymph nodes.[31]

There is a depression of delayed hypersensitivity as manifested by skin testing to a variety of antigens. This suggests a T-lymphocyte-mediated anergy and impaired cellular immunity. The granuloma formation which occurs in this disease may be due to a macrophage migration inhibition factor liberated from T-lymphocytes of patients with sarcoidosis. This is thought to be the basis of the Kveim test, in which the skin of patients with sarcoidosis reacts to an injection of a suspension of sarcoid tissue by developing a localized granuloma.

In contrast to the depressed cellular immunity, there appears to be either normal or overactive function of the humoral immune response.[32] Elevated levels of IgG, IgA, and IgM have been reported in sarcoidosis. The meaning of these immune abnormalities remains unclear.

IMMUNODEFICIENCY UVEITIS (OPPORTUNISTIC UVEITIDES)

As a result of new treatment regimens such as renal dialysis, cancer chemotherapy, and organ transplantation, patients so treated may manifest ocular disease in two different ways: 1) entirely new conditions not previously encountered; 2) bizarre and exaggerated findings in older, recognized entities.

These eye problems are seen in patients who have been exogenously (cytotoxic drugs or steroids) or endogenously immunosuppressed (lymphoid malignan-

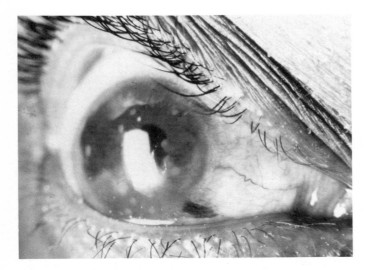

Figure 8.4 Sarcoidosis with granulomata of the iris.

cies, widespread metastatic disease, or congenital or acquired immunodeficiency states such as uremia). The eye diseases result from low resistance to infection with subsequent infection by traditionally nonpathogenic organisms. The introduction of antibiotics had a profound influence in decreasing the incidence and severity of metastatic bacterial endophthalmitis which had virtually disappeared. With the emergence of this immunosuppressed or immunodeficient group of patients, we have begun to see a new form of uveitis or metastatic endophthalmitis caused by nonpathogenic or opportunistic organisms. These include the fungi, *Candida* (Fig. 8.5), *Aspergillus*, and *Cryptococcus*;[33] herpes viruses, including herpes simplex iridocyclitis and retinitis, herpes zoster iridocyclitis,[34] and the cytomegalovirus, with more retinal than uveal involvement;[35] subacute sclerosing panencephalitis secondary to measles; an indolent type of metastatic endophthalmitis caused by staphylococcal organisms;[37] and ocular toxoplasmosis, which is seen more frequently in patients immunosuppressed by Hodgkin's disease[38] (Fig. 8.6).

Inflammatory and immune responses are impaired by both endogenous and exogenous types of immunosuppression. This depression of the immune response is probably responsible for the initial spread of an organism and the lack of subsequent severe inflammation. The

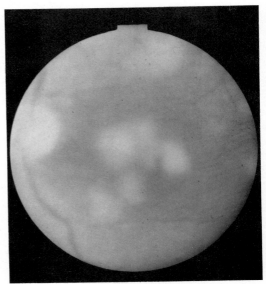

Figure 8.5 Metastatic endophthalmitis due to *Candida albicans* in an immunosuppressed renal patient.

nonpathogenic nature of the infecting organism also helps explain the often indolent nature of these low grade inflammatory processes.

Ophthalmologists must be aware of these new clinical populations and their new and altered eye problems. The patient with a metastatic endophthalmitis secondary to one of these organisms might complain of only slight blurring of vision or floaters instead of a painful red eye. A history of stress may often be elicited from

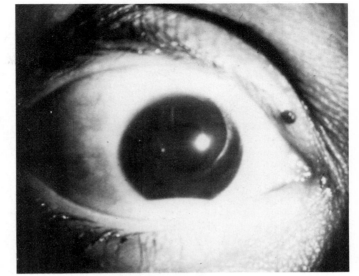

Figure 8.6 Hypopyon in a minimally injected eye of an immunosuppressed patient with presumed staphylococcal endophthalmitis.

otherwise healthy patients with recurrent uveitis. This suggests that, as in the case of herpes, the patient becomes self-immunosuppressed by raising his own production of 17-hydroxycorticosteroids. This may allow the temporary emergence of an organism and subsequent infection with a response manifested as uveitis. The important point is that the stress may result in temporary immunosuppression.

This simple and facile hypothesis, although interesting, requires scientific validation. It has been stated that one-fourth of patients with ocular histoplasmosis relate both the onset and frequency of repeated episodes of macular involvement to emotional stress.[39]

REFERENCES

1. Prisnow, J.F., Hall, J.M. Studies on intravitreal initiation of the immune response. Invest. Ophthalmol. 9:639–646, 1970.
2. Silverstein, A.M., Zimmerman, L.F. Immunogenic endophthalmitis produced in the guinea pig by different pathogenetic mechanisms. Am. J. Ophthalmol. 48:435–447, 1959.
3. Bloch-Michel, E. Uveitis by humoral flood or medicine allergy. In Uveitis: Immunologic and Allergic Phenomena, edited by Campinchi, R., Faure, J.P., Bloch-Michel, E., and Haut, J., Charles C Thomas, Springfield, 1973, pp. 315–321.
4. Friedlaender, M.H. Allergy and Immunology of the Eye. Harper and Row, Hagerstown, 1979, p. 43.
5. Theodore, F.H., Lewson, A.C. Bilateral iritis complicating serum sickness. Arch. Ophthalmol. 21:828–832, 1939.
6. Sedan, J., Guillot, P. Uvéities medicamenteuses. Bull. et mém. Soc. franc d'opht. 11:145, 1955.
7. O'Connor, G.R. Recurrent herpes simplex uveitis in humans. Surv. Ophthalmol. 21:165–170, 1976.
8. Spaeth, G.C. Absence of so-called histoplasma uveitis in 134 cases of proven histoplasmosis. Arch. Ophthalmol. 77:41, 1967.
9. Krause, A.C., Hopkins, W.G. Ocular manifestations of histoplasmosis. Am. J. Ophthalmol. 34:564, 1951.
10. Schirmer, O: IX International Congress Ophthalmology Utrecht 402, 1899.
11. Verhoeff, F., Lemoine, A.N. Hypersensitiveness to lens protein. Am. J. Ophthalmol. 5:700, 1922.
12. Breinin, G.M. Danger of fish lens protein injection as treatment for cataract. J. Am. Med. Assoc. 152:698–700, 1953.
13. Posner, A. Complications following injection of fish lens protein for cataract. J. Am. Med. Assoc. 151:317, 1953.
14. Marak, G.E., Font, R.L., Alepa, F.P. Experimental lens induced granulomatous endophthalmitis. Mod. Probl. Ophthalmol. 16:75–79, 1976.
14a. Marak, G.E., Font, R.L., Alepa, F.P. Immunopathogenicity of lens crystallins in the production of experimental lens-induced granulomatous endophthalmitis. Ophthalmol. Res. 10:30–35, 1978.
15. Blodi, F.C. Sympathetic uveitis as an allergic phenomenon. Trans. Am. Acad. Ophthalmol. Otolarynol. 63:642–649, 1959.
16. Elschnig, A. Zur Frage der sympatischen Ophthalmie. Klin. Monatsbl. Augenheilkd.

80:289, 1928.

17. Woods, A.C. Diseases of the uvea. Sympathetic ophthalmia I. The use of uveal pigment in diagnosis and treatment. Trans. Ophthalmol. Soc. UK 45:208, 1925.

18. Friedenwald, J.S. Notes on the allergy theory of sympathetic ophthalmia. Am. J. Ophthalmol. 17:1008–1018, 1934.

19. Collins, R.C. Further experimental studies on sympathetic ophthalmia. Am. J. Ophthalmol. 36:150–162,1953.

20. Naquin, H.A. An unsuccessful attempt to produce hypersensitivity to uveal tissue in guinea pigs. Am. J. Ophthalmol. 39:196–200, 1955.

21. Aronson, S.B., McMaster, P.R.B. Passive transfer of experimental allergic uveitis. Arch. Ophthalmol. 86:557, 1971.

22. Marak, G.E., Jr., Aye, M.S., Alepa, F.P. Cellular hypersensitivity in penetrating eye injuries. Invest. Ophthalmol. 12:380, 1973.

23. Marak, G.E., Jr., Font, R.L., Johnson, M.C., Alepa, F.P. Lymphocyte-stimulating activity of ocular tissues in sympathetic ophthalmia. Invest. Ophthalmol. 10:770, 1971.

24. Wacker, W.B.: Experimental allergic uveitis. Int. Arch. Allergy 45:639, 1973.

24a. Nussenblatt, R.B., Rodriques, M.M., Salinas-Carmona, M.C., Gery, I., Cevario, S., Wacker, W. Modulation of experimental autoimmune uveitis with cyclosporin A. Arch. Ophthalmol. 100:1146–1149, 1982.

24b. Nussenblatt, R.B., Mittal, K.K., Ryan, S., Green, W.R., Maumenee, A.E. Birdshot retinochoroidopathy associated with HLA-A29 antigen and immune responsiveness to retinal S-antigen. Am. J. Ophthalmol. 94:147–158, 1982.

25. Hammer, H: Cellular hypersensitivity to uveal pigment confirmed by leukocyte migration tests in sympathetic ophthalmitis and the Vogt-Koyanagi-Harada syndrome. Br. J. Ophthalmol. 58:773, 1974.

26. Behcet, H. Uber rezidivierende, aphthöse, durch ein Virus verursachte Geschwüre am Mund, am Auge und an den Genitalien. Dermatol. Woch-enschr. 105:1152–1157, 1937.

27. Theodore, F.H. Ocular-oral syndromes. Oral Surg. 5:259–270, 1952.

28. Lehner, T., Barnes, C.G. (eds.) Behcet's Syndrome: Clinical and Immunological Features. Academic Press, New York, 1980.

29. Gupta, R.C., O'Duffy, J.D., McDuffie, F.C., Meuer, M., Jordon, R.E. Circulating immune complexes in active Behcet's disease. Clin. Exp. Immunol. 34:213–218, 1978.

30. James, D.G. Uveitis—immunopathy or infection? Trans. Ophthalmol. Soc. UK, 88:711–727, 1968.

31. Tannenbaum, H., Rocklin, R.E., Schur, P.H., Shetter, A.L. Immune function in sarcoidosis studies on delayed hypersensitivity. B and T lymphocytes, serum immunoglobulins and serum complement components. Clin. Exp. Immunol. 26:511, 1976.

32. Patnode, R.A., Allin, R.C., Carpenter, R.L. Serum immunoglobulin levels in sarcoidosis. Am. J. Clin. Pathol. 45:398–401, 1966.

33. Char, D.H. Immunology of Uveitis and Ocular Tumors. Grune and Stratton, New York, 1978, p. 69.

34. Bloom, J.N., Katz, J.I., Kaufman, H.E. Herpes simplex retinitis and encephalitis in an adult. Arch. Ophthalmol. 95:1798, 1977.

35. Cogan, D.G.: Immunosuppression and eye disease. Am. J. Ophthalmol. 83:777, 1977.

36. Zimmerman, L.E. Changing concepts concerning the pathogenesis of infectious diseases. Am. J. Ophthalmol. 69:947–964, 1970.

37. Bloomfield, S.E., David, D.S., Cheigh, J.S., Kim, Y., White, R.P., Stenzel, K.H., Rubin, A.L. Endophthalmitis following staphylococcal sepsis in renal failure patients. Arch. Intern. Med. 138:706–708, 1978.

38. O'Connor, G.R. Uveitis in the immunocompromised host. N. Engl. J. Med. 299:130–132, 1978.

39. Gass, J.D., Wilkinson, C.P. Follow-up study of presumed ocular histoplasmosis. Trans. Am. Acad. Ophthalmol. Otolaryngol. 76:672, 1972.

CHAPTER NINE

Retina and Optic Nerve

The retinal pigment epithelium and photoreceptor outer segments are now known to be active metabolic structures. In addition, several investigators have shown experimentally that both of these structures are antigenic and can produce humoral and cell-mediated responses.[1-3] As mentioned in the previous chapter, several authors feel that the problem in sympathetic ophthalmia is autoimmune but the antigen is retinal, not uveal. Table 9.1 lists immune disorders of the retina and optic nerve.

Hypersensitivity versus Hyperreactivity

In evaluating reactions occurring in the retina and optic nerve, a distinction must be made between allergy and hyperreactivity, especially in regard to drugs. Everyone accepts the fact that when poisons are taken in large enough or toxic doses, tissue death will result. It is generally not realized, however, that in certain hyperreactive individuals, minute amounts of the same drug may cause a similar reaction. It should be clear that this is not allergy, because the person so affected reacts in a manner only quantitatively different from that of the average person. For example, most people would react to large doses of atropine taken internally with the classic pharmacological and toxic effects, such as vomiting, tachycardia, fever, and dilatation of the pupil. When, however, an individual reacts in the same manner, with the same symptoms, after injection of a very small amount of atropine, or reacts similarly after its local instillation into the eye, this is in a sense a toxic effect following a minute dose, or hyperreactivity. In other words, the only difference in the reaction here is a quantitative one in regard to dosage. In contrast, when a person is allergic or hypersensitive to a drug, the response involves entirely different symptoms, essentially allergic in character. These include asthma, rhinitis, urticaria, skin eruptions, and other accepted allergic phenomena. These are not the pharmacological effects of the drug. Moreover, when they do occur they are the same regardless of which particular drug the patient has used. Other examples of hyperreactivity important to the ophthalmologist are quinine amblyopia and reactions occurring with minute amounts of nicotine or following the use of atropine and cocaine. Marked ciliary spasms from extremely small amounts of pilocarpine and other miotics should also be noted.

RETINA

Atopic Reactions

Most instances of proven neuroretinal allergy have occurred in the course of serum sickness. Now that antisera are used less frequently, such occurrences are encountered far less often. There have been reported cases of neuroretinitis resulting from allergy to such foods as peanuts, fish, chocolate, milk, eggs, and cola. Pollens such as primrose and ragweed have also been incriminated. Sulfonamides, penicillin, and procaine have been observed to give rise to allergic retinal reactions (Fig. 9.1). Generalized angioedema due to a variety of agents has resulted in retinal exudative lesions. Instances of retrobulbar neuritis occurring on the basis of atopic allergic reactions, usually due to foods, also have been reported.[4]

Table 9.1
Clinical Reactions of the Retina and Optic Nerve

Retina
1. Atopic and anaphylactic reactions—serum, food, pollen, drugs, angioneurotic edema and urticaria
2. Microbiallergic reactions
   a. *Toxocara*, toxoplasmosis
3. Retinal vasculitis
   a. Eales' disease
   b. Polyarteritis nodosa
   c. Central retinal vein thrombosis
4. Autoimmune
   a. Retinitis pigmentosa (?)
   b. Macular degeneration (?)
   c. Sympathetic ophthalmia
5. Immunodeficiency retinitis (or opportunistic retinitis)
   a. Immunosuppressed patients—cytomegalic virus, herpes simplex virus, diffuse toxoplasmosis
   b. Immunoimmature patients—newborn rubella, herpes simplex virus
Optic Nerve
1. Autoimmune—multiple sclerosis
2. Hypersensitivity reactions—tobacco-alcohol amblyopia

Microbiallergic Reactions

Infection of the retina, as in the uvea, may arise secondarily to both pathogenic or nonpathogenic organisms, depending on the clinical situation. In normal or immunocompetent patients, we may see not only the infection, but also a hypersensitivity or microbiallergic reaction to the offending organism. In an immune compromised patient, infection by nonpathogenic organisms can result in retinal damage. This is not a microbiallergic reaction. Indeed, there is an underreactivity of response to the organism, not a hypersensitivity.

Even though instances of microbiallergic neuroretinitis are rare, a number of rather convincing cases have been reported. Weizenblatt[5] described such a reaction occurring on two occasions in a patient with marked cutaneous sensitivity to old tuberculin, 5 to 7 days after skin testing with this antigen. Other reports describe similar exudative retinitis from tuberculin injections and in trypanosomiasis.[4] Retrobulbar neuritis has resulted from prophylactic vaccination against rabies.

Retinal hypersensitivity reactions may occur with pathogenic organisms such as *Toxocara canis*. This usually occurs in children, taking the form of a unilateral retinal granuloma, with fibrinoid necrosis, eosinophils, lymphocytes, and plasma cell infiltration around a toxocara larva incarcerated in a branch of the retinal artery. There may be a more extensive exudative endophthalmitis. As in other systemic helminth infestations, the immunological response to *T. canis* is characterized by increased levels of circulating IgE and blood eosinophilia. The presence of IgE antibodies forms the basis for a skin test which can be used in the diagnosis.[6, 7] The introduction of an enzyme-linked immunosorbent assay (ELISA) for *T. canis* antibody has helped in the diagnosis of ocular Toxocariasis because it is more sensitive than previously available tests. ELISA titers can be demonstrated in aqueous and vitreous samples at higher levels than those in sera, suggesting localized antibody production to *T. canis* in the eye.[8, 9]

Toxoplasmosis in the immunocompetent host results in a characteristic focal necrotizing retinitis. It is postulated that the initial ocular lesion results from invasion of the retinal cells by rapidly multiplying organisms which then enter a cystic phase in a subsiding inflammatory lesion. The recurrent attacks of toxoplasmosis retinochoroiditis are thought to be due to rupture of the cysts or a hypersensitivity reaction to *Toxoplasma* antigen or autoantigens. A recent study of a monkey model of ocular toxoplasmosis suggested that hypersensitivity to *Toxoplasma* antigens does not play a major role in triggering recurrences of toxoplasmic retinochoroiditis in nonhuman primates.[9a] Infection by this organism results in the production of IgG and IgM antibodies, detectable by serological techniques. However, the presence of antibody does not protect the host from infection. The chief defense against this organism is through the cell-mediated immune mechanism and the T-lymphocyte-macrophage axis.[10, 11] Drugs suppressing this immunity, such as corticosteroids and cytotoxic agents, in the past used to treat the ocular inflammation in this disease, can also lead to dissemination of the parasite.[12] This is why we see more diffuse toxoplasmosis in the immunosuppressed patient.

Retinal Vasculitis

An inflammatory involvement of retinal vessels occurs in numerous conditions, with or without systemic involvement. Eales' disease, a primary retinal vasculitis or periphlebitis, occurs in adolescents and young men and is often bilateral. The disease affects mainly peripheral retinal vessels, but a less common variant involves larger veins of the posterior fundus. The involved vessels are sheathed in a lymphocytic exudate and are liable to thrombose with subsequent hemorrhage, preretinal neovascularization, and scar formation. Lymphocytes predominate, but plasma cells may also be seen. Serum levels of IgG and IgA have been reported raised in Eales' disease.[13] Chilman,[14] in 1973, found increased amounts of IgM, as well as autoantibodies to cell nuclei, mitochondria, and smooth muscle cells in some patients. There may be initial vascular damage caused by an exogenous agent with subsequent changes attributable to an autoallergic response to altered tissue antigens.

Retinal vessels are affected in some generalized connective tissue disorders, such as polyarteritis nodosa and systemic lupus erythematosus. In these situations, it is believed that immune complex deposition in the retinal vessels plays a strong role in the findings in the posterior fundus.[15]

A variant of central retinal vein thrombosis occurs in a younger group of patients. Lyle and Wybar, in 1961,[16] suggested that the disturbance in these cases is mainly a phlebitis, rather than a thrombosis.

In summary, some of the retinal vas-

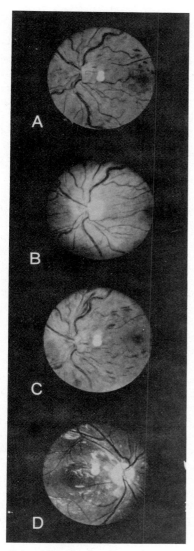

Figure 9.1 Allergic fundus reactions. *A*, Petechial hemorrhages in a patient sensitive to procaine. *B*, same patient after resorption. *C*, recurrence 2 months later following another injection of procaine. *D*, allergic edema of nerve head and retina due to tetanus antitoxin. (Reprinted with permission from Bedell, A.J. J. Am. Med. Assoc. 105:1502, 1935.)

cular diseases (such as Eales' disease) which occur alone or vascular disease seen in collagen problems and variations of central vein thrombosis may be due to an immunogenic inflammation.

Retinal Degenerations—Possible Autoimmunity

The finding that the retinal pigment epithelium and photoreceptor outer segments are antigenic raises intriguing questions concerning the pathophysiology of some of the so-called degenerative retinal diseases. The cause of degeneration of the retinal pigment epithelium and photoreceptors in retinitis pigmentosa remains a mystery. While several investigators have emphasized the possible role of the pigment epithelium in retinitis pigmentosa,[17, 18] this hypothesis remains to be proven. Macular degeneration has been shown to result in the accumulation of macrophages. But it remains to be seen whether they are present in response to dying tissue or as an inciting stimulus to the disease process. Therefore, the concept of an autoimmune etiology in these entities remains a hypothesis since the evidence is largely indirect and not entirely persuasive. But it is an interesting and fresh approach to a difficult problem.

Immunodeficiency Retinitis (Opportunistic Retinitis)

In the immunosuppressed patient, the immune imbalance lies on the host side, so that normally nonpathogenic organisms are allowed to take hold, resulting in tissue damage. As many diseases are now being treated with immunosuppressive drugs, the emergence of new retinal problems can be expected (described in Chapter Eight). Infections with cytomegalic virus, herpes simplex virus, and a more diffuse type of toxoplasmic retinochoroiditis are being seen in patients who are immunosuppressed both from an underlying disease and by immunosuppressive drugs used in treatment. The tissue damage from these organisms is a direct consequence of their replication within the infected cells and not the body's immune reaction against them. The damage is due to the absence of a protective immunological mechanism, and is not the result of cell-mediated hypersensitivity against the organism. Therefore, the organism is not causing any immune inflammation, but the lack of host defense results in infection. Indeed, that is why these infections are often indolent and show little inflammation. Tissue damage may result without signs of florid reactions. In immunoimmature patients, such as the newborn, one sees a similar type of infestation, often of nonpathogenic organisms. Rubella virus and herpes simplex may cause diffuse inflammation of the retina with subsequent pigmentation. Infants lack a strong immune response to viral antigens in the first few months of life. The natural killer cell seems to be responsible for clearing viral infections. The natural killer cell is very low in cord blood during the first few months of life.[19]

OPTIC NERVE

The optic nerve consists of myelinated nerve fibers and supporting glial tissue. The protein myelin has been shown to be capable of provoking an immune response, such as an allergic encephalomyelitis, when injected subcutaneously into normal animals.[20] Multiple sclerosis (MS), the most important cause of an optic neuritis, is suspected of having an autoimmune basis, because of both its similarity to chronic experimental allergic optic neuritis and of other immunological data. Antibodies to myelin are present in the serum of most patients, and can be correlated with active phases of the disease.[21, 22] Optic neuritis might also result after certain viral infections and vaccination procedures. A virus may play a role as an initiating factor, with the subsequent tissue damage being caused by an autoimmune phenomenon. In addition, there is a prevalence of HLA-Dw2 in MS patients.[23] The etiology of toxic amblyopias remains to be determined. The question arises, is this a hyperreactivity to small quantities of foreign materials or a true allergic reaction? In tobacco-alcohol amblyopia, some intriguing work suggests that a tobacco allergen which has been purified and shown to be a glycoprotein may activate Hageman factor, thus initiating the clotting sequence resulting in thrombosis.[24] If this tobacco glycoprotein results in thrombosis of small vessels around the optic nerve, it could result in a so-called toxic amblyopia, which is ultimately caused by a tobacco allergen initiating the clotting sequence.

REFERENCES

1. Marak, G.E., Jr., Aye, M.S., Alepa, F.P. Cellular hypersensitivity in penetrating eye injuries. Invest. Ophthalmol. 12:380, 1973.
2. Wong, V.G., Green, W.R., Kuwabara, T., McMaster, P.R.B., Cameron, T.P. Homologous retinal outer segment immunization in primates. Arch. Ophthalmol. 93:509, 1975.
3. Reich D'Almeida, F., Rahi, A.H.S. Antigenic specificity of retinal pigment epithelium and non-immunological involvement in retinal dystrophy. Nature 252:307–308, 1974.
4. Theodore, F.H., Schlossman, A. Ocular Allergy. Williams & Wilkins, Baltimore, 1958.
5. Weizenblatt, S. Allergic ocular reactions to the tuberculin test: Bilateral cyclitis and neuroretinitis. Arch. Ophthalmol. 41:436–443, 1949.
6. Brown, D.H.: Ocular toxocara. I. Experimental immunology. Ann. Ophthalmol. 3:907, 1970.
7. Brown, D.H. Ocular toxocara. II. Clinical review. J. Ped. Ophthalmol. 7:182, 1970.
8. Biglan, A.W., Glickman, L.T., Lobes, L. A. Serum and vitreous Toxocara antibody in nematode endophthalmitis. Am. J. Ophthalmol. 88:898–901, 1979.
9. Felberg, N.T., Shields, J.A., Federman, J.L. Antibody to Toxocara canis in the aqueous humor. Arch. Ophthalmol. 99:1563–1564, 1981.
9a. Newman, P.E., Ghosheh, R., Tabbara, K.F., O'Connor, G.R., Stern, W.: The role of hypersensitivity reactions to Toxoplasma antigens in experimental ocular toxoplasmosis in nonhuman primates. Am. J. Ophthalmol. 94:159–164, 1982.
10. Borges, J.S., Johnson, W.D., Jr. Inhibition of multiplication of Toxoplasma gondii by human monocytes exposed to T lymphocyte products. J. Exp. Med. 141:483, 1975.
11. Jones, T.C., Len L., Hirsch, J.G. Assessment in vitro of immunity against Toxoplasma gondii. J. Exp. Med. 141:466, 1975.
12. O'Connor, G.R., Frenkel, J.K. Dangers of steroid treatment in toxoplasmosis. Arch. Ophthalmol. 94:213, 1976.
13. Johnson, G.J., Bloch, K.K. Immunoglobulin levels in retinal vascular abnormalities and pseudoxanthoma elasticum. Arch. Ophthalmol. 81:322, 1969.
14. Chilman, T. Specific and non-specific antibody activity in retinal vasculitis. Trans. Ophthalmol. Soc. UK 93:193, 1973.
15. Agnello, V., Koffler, D., Eisenberg, J.W., Winchester, R.J., Kunkel, H.G. C1q precipitins in the sera of patients with systemic lupus erythematosus and other hypo-complementemic states: characterization of high and some low molecular weights. J. Exp. Med. 134:2285, 1971.
16. Lyle, K.T., Wybar, K. Retinal vasculitis. Br. J. Ophthalmol. 45:787–788, 1961.
17. Feeney, L. The phagolysosomal system of the pigment-epithelium: A key to retinal disease. Invest. Ophthalmol. 12:635–638, 1973.
18. Burden, E.M., Yates, C.M., Reading, H.W. Investigation into the structural integrity of lysosomes in the normal and dystrophic rat retina. Exp. Eye Res. 12:159–165, 1972.
19. Lopez, C. Unpublished data.
20. Kies, M.W., Alvord, E.C. Encephalitogenic activity in guinea pigs of water soluble protein fractions of nervous tissue. In Allergic Encephalitis, edited by Kies, M.W., and Alvord, E.C. Charles C Thomas, Springfield, 1959, pp. 293–299.
21. Lumsden, C.E. The immunogenesis of the multiple sclerosis plaque. Brain Res. 28:365–390, 1971.
22. Bornstein, M. Immunopathology of the demyelinative disorders: tissue culture studies. In Immunopathology, Fourth International Symposium, edited by Grabar, P., and Miescher, P. Schwabe, Basel, 1966, pp. 374–391.
23. Platz, P., Ryder, L.P., Nielsen, L., Svejgaard, A., Thomsen, M., Wolheim, M.S. HL-A and idiopathic optic neuritis. Lancet 1:520, 1975.
24. Becker, C.G., Dubin, T. Activation of factor XII by tobacco glycoprotein. J. Exp. Med. 146:457–467, 1977.

CHAPTER TEN

The Orbit and Lacrimal Gland

Unlike the eye itself, the orbit does not contain any antigenically unique tissue. Even the lacrimal gland is antigenically similar to the extraorbital salivary glands. Therefore, the orbit would not be expected to manifest any immunological disorders peculiar to itself. It can be involved in generalized disorders such as the connective tissue diseases, as is outlined in previous chapters. However, there are some orbital conditions which should be mentioned.

ALLERGIC ORBITAL EDEMA

Since any orbital swelling in the confines of the bony cavity will result in anterior dislocation of the globe and dramatic proptosis, even minor degrees of edema can produce striking effects. Allergic orbital edema can complicate anaphylactic hypersensitivity reactions affecting the lids or conjunctiva and may be a feature of heredity angioneurotic edema in which there is a congenital defect of C1 inhibitor. It has been speculated that a transient but recurrent form of proptosis, appearing spontaneously in some individuals, may be an expression of allergic edema. Edema of the lids, seen in serum sickness and some drug and food allergies due to type III or IV hypersensitivity, may spill over into the orbit.[1]

THYROID EXOPHTHALMOS

The main basis for the proptosis in thyroid exophthalmos is an increase in orbital fat and mucopolysaccharides. In addition, the extraocular muscles are swollen and diffusely infiltrated with lympho-cytes and plasma cells. The direct cause of the increased orbital connective tissues is under active investigation. The exophthalmos associated with thyroid dysfunction is currently attributed to exophthalmos producing substance (EPS), which represents fragments of the thyroid stimulating hormones (TSH) secreted by the pituitary. Binding of these TSH fragments to orbital tissue is facilitated by an IgG autoantibody.[2] There is some evidence that the increase in mucopolysaccharide and consequent retention of fluid is a direct effect of the antibody bound TSH fragments on the orbital connective tissues.[3] An increase in orbital fat is also said to occur in possible response to TSH fragments. Another hormone called long-acting thyroid stimulator (LATS) has a stimulating effect on orbital fat.

LATS is an IgG autoantibody that is probably directed against antigen on the thyroid cell surface. When LATS binds to thyroid cells, it stimulates a constant production of T-4 hormone.[4] LATS has an effect similar to that of TSH, but it is not under the control of the thyroid-pituitary axis. This is an example of what is called "stimulatory hypersensitivity" or a type V reaction.[5] An inflammatory edema is also involved in the extraocular muscles. This is mediated by immune complex deposition with consequent activation of complement and release of vasoactive amines. Why immune complexes should accumulate in the orbit is not known.[6]

MYASTHENIA GRAVIS

The ocular symptoms of myasthenia gravis (MG) include external ophthalmoplegia, paresis of accommodation, inadequate convergence, and diplopia. Because of coexistence with other disorders having an autoimmune basis, especially thyroid disease and pernicious anemia, and because of its common association with thymic pathology, MG has been suspected of having an autoimmune basis for some years. The affected muscles show acute necrotizing inflammation with progressive atrophy and focal lymphocyte infiltration around degenerating muscle fibers. Specific IgG antibodies to skeletal muscle have been found.[7] These antibodies were demonstrated against acetylcholine receptor protein in the serum of as many as 87% of patients with MG. This and other evidence suggests that MG involves an antibody-mediated autoimmune attack on acetylcholine receptors at the neuromuscular junction.[8]

It is of interest that thymus abnormalities are present in 80% of myasthenic patients. Some 70% have thymic hyperplasia, and 10% have true thymomas. The thymus gland, which plays such an important role in the development of the T-lymphocyte, shows increased numbers of B-lymphocytes in hyperplastic thymuses examined from patients with MG. Two-thirds of patients who undergo thymectomy have complete or partial remission of MG, suggesting that the thymus may be a site for production of a neuromuscular blocking agent.[9] The role, if any, of

cellular immunity remains unclear and under investigation.

LYMPHOPROLIFERATIVE DISORDERS OF THE ORBIT

The infiltration of the orbit with lymphocytes can present a practical problem on how to distinguish between a non-neoplastic lymphocytic proliferation (such as reactive follicular hyperplasia or inflammatory pseudotumor) and the more serious infiltrations of malignant lymphomas.[10] There are some lymphocyte infiltrations that seem to occupy an intermediate position between a lymphoid pseudotumor and a lymphoma. The etiology of these obscure infiltrations remains unknown (Fig. 10.1).

Recent advances in immunological techniques may enable us to differentiate more accurately between these three entities. The lymphoid cell populations can be studied by their cell surface markers to determine if they are all T- or all B-lymphocytes (monoclonal), or a mixture of both (polyclonal).

It is postulated that benign lesions are polyclonal and that malignant orbital lymphoid proliferations are monoclonal. The cell surface marker data must be correlated with the histopathology and interpreted within the clinical setting of each patient.[11]

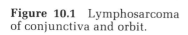

Figure 10.1 Lymphosarcoma of conjunctiva and orbit.

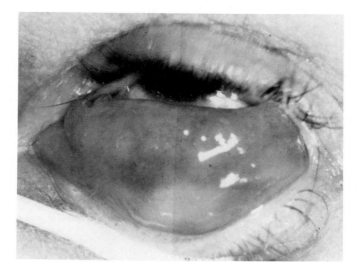

SJÖGREN'S SYNDROME

Sjögren's syndrome is characterized by the triad of keratoconjunctivitis sicca, xerostomia and rheumatoid arthritis, or another connective tissue disease. The presence of two of these three conditions is generally considered sufficient for the diagnosis.[12, 13] Criteria for the diagnosis of Sjögren's syndrome in other studies include dry eyes, dry mouth, and a biopsy of the minor salivary glands of the lip showing lymphoid infiltration.[14] The combination of keratoconjunctivitis sicca and xerostomia in itself is sometimes referred to as the sicca syndrome.

Sjögren's syndrome has an insidious onset and usually occurs in middle age. Over 90% of the patients are female. Patients may complain of dry mouth due to salivary gland hyposecretion. They also complain of difficulty in chewing or swallowing food. Parotid gland enlargement occurs in approximately 50% of patients. Drying of the nasal mucosa may lead to recurrent epistaxis, and drying of the larynx may lead to hoarseness.

Patients with Sjögren's syndrome develop keratoconjunctivitis sicca from deficient aqueous tear secretion of the lacrimal glands. They complain of ocular irritation, redness, foreign body sensation, itching, burning, and photophobia. They may also report a lack of tears in response to emotional stimuli. Clinical examination reveals conjunctival hyperemia and edema and erythema of the lid margins. Corneal filaments may be found. Superficial punctate staining with fluorescein is found on the cornea and bulbar conjunctiva, especially in the interpalpebral region. Mucous debris may be found in the tear film. Tear film break up times may be rapid, and Schirmer tear volumes are usually less than 5 mm. Tear lysozyme levels are deficient or absent in this condition. Keratinized epithelial cells can usually be demonstrated by Giemsa stain of conjunctival scrapings. Corneal complications of Sjögren's syndrome include vascularization, ulceration, scarring, and even perforation.

Immunopathology

Patients with Sjögren's syndrome develop lymphoid infiltration of the lacrimal and salivary glands that results in glandular tissue destruction with permanent scarring and fibrosis.[12] Both T and B-lymphocytes have been detected in the salivary gland infiltrates.[15]

Hypergammaglobulinemia usually of the polyclonal-type is a frequent finding in Sjögren's syndrome. Rheumatoid factor and antinuclear antibodies are found in the majority of patients with Sjögren's syndrome.[15]

In one study, antibodies to salivary duct cells were found in 16 of 30 patients (53%) with Sjögren's syndrome.[13] The antibodies were IgG and IgM, but rarely IgA. One-third of the antibodies were complement-fixing. The antibodies to salivary duct cells could only be absorbed with salivary gland tissue and not with other tissues. Antinuclear factor was demonstrated in 77% of the sera, rheumatoid factor in 48%, and antibodies to smooth muscle in 19%. Antibodies to skeletal muscle, gastric parietal cells, thyroid antigens, adrenal cortex, and mitochondria were found in frequencies which did not differ significantly from those in matched controls. The lymphocytes of patients with Sjögren's syndrome show impaired transformation in response to mitogens and impaired delayed hypersensitivity to a specific contact allergen.[16] Cellular hypersensitivity to salivary gland extracts has been demonstrated in patients with Sjögren's syndrome using peripheral blood lymphocytes.[12]

Sjögren's syndrome is associated with HLA-B 8. HLA-Dw3, a lymphocyte-defined determinant known to be in strong linkage disequilibrium with HLA-B 8, was studied in patients with Sjögren's syndrome.[14] It was found that the primary association of Sjögren's syndrome was with HLA-Dw3 which was observed in 84% of patients with Sjögren's syndrome in the absence of rheumatoid arthritis, compared to 24% in controls. The frequency of HLA-B 8 and HLA-Dw3 in patients with both Sjögren's syndrome and rheumatoid arthritis did not differ from that in controls. It was concluded that patients with Sjögren's syndrome alone and those with Sjögren's syndrome and rheumatoid arthritis comprise genetically distinct groups.

Patients with Sjögren's syndrome have

a predisposition to develop lympho-proliferative disorders.[12] These include lymphomas, reticulum cell sarcoma, and Waldenstrom's macroglobulinemia.

The hybrid of New Zealand black and New Zealand white mice was found to develop characteristic findings of Sjögren's syndrome in salivary tissue in addition to a disease resembling systemic lupus erythematosus.[17, 18] The cornea and conjunctiva showed changes compatible with Sjögren's syndrome in humans. The Gross leukemia virus was found in these mice. The autoimmune findings in these mice appear to involve an interaction of genetic, immunological, and viral factors.[12]

Treatment

An associated connective tissue disease should be treated with systemic corticosteroids or immunosuppressives, if necessary. For the oral manifestations, it is important for the patient to maintain good oral hygiene with regular dental examinations and frequent use of mouth washes. Management of dry eye includes the use of artificial tears, a humid environment, goggles, plastic shields, and occlusion of the lacrimal puncta. Recently, alternate day therapy with systemic corticosteroids was found to inhibit the mononuclear cell infiltration of accessory salivary glands and to improve both the signs and symptoms of keratoconjunctivitis sicca in patients with Sjögren's syndrome.[19] There was an improvement in corneal staining, a decrease in corneal filaments, an increase in Schirmer tear volumes, an increase in tear lysozyme levels and a reduction of the mononuclear cell infiltration of accessory salivary glands in patients receiving alternate day systemic corticosteroids. Bromhexine which is used for treating chronic bronchitis has been found to increase lysozyme levels in patients with keratoconjunctivitis sicca and systemic diseases and, to a lesser degree, in patients with keratoconjunctivitis sicca only.[20] It also relieves ocular symptoms and improves Schirmer test findings in some patients.

REFERENCES

1. Rahi, A.H.S., Garner, A. The orbit. In Immunopathology of the Eye. Blackwell, Oxford, 1976, p. 239.
2. Doniach, D., Roitt, I.M. Thyroid auto-allergic disease. In Clinical Aspects of Immunology, edited by Gell, P.G.H., Coombs, R.R.A., Lachmann, P.J., 3rd ed. Blackwell, Oxford, 1975, pp. 1355–1386.
3. Lavergne, G., Winand, R. L'exophtalmie endocrinienne. Bull. Soc. belge Ophthal 163:1–170, 1973.
4. Hart, I.R., McKenzie, J.M. Comparison of the effects of thyrotropin and long-acting thyroid stimulator on guinea-pig adipose tissue. Endocrinology 88:26–30, 1971.
5. Roitt, I.M. Essential Immunology, ed. 2 Blackwell, Oxford, 1975.
6. Komishi, J., Herman, M.M., Kriss, J.P. Binding of thyroglobulin and thyroglobulin antithyroglobulin immune-complexes to extraocular muscles membrane. Endocrinology 95:434–446, 1974.
7. Irvine, W.J., Kalden, J.R. Muscle in allergic disease. In Clinical Aspects of Immunology, ed. 3 edited by Gell, P.G.H., Coombs, R.R.A., and Lachman, P.J. Blackwell, Oxford, 1975, pp. 1467–1507.
8. Bender, A.N., Ringel, S.P., Engel, W.K., Daniels, M.P., Vogel, Z. Myasthenia gravis: A serum factor blocking acetylcholine receptors of the human neuromuscular junction. Lancet 1:607, 1975.
9. Friedlaender, M. Neurologic and endocrine diseases. In Allergy and Immunology of the Eye. Harper and Row, Hagerstown, 1979, p. 275.
10. Knowles, D., Jakobiec, F. Orbital lymphoid neoplasms: Clinical, pathologic and immunologic characteristics. In Ocular and Adnexal Tumors. Aesculapius, Birmingham, 1978, pp. 806–838.
11. Knowles, D.M., Jakobiec, F., Halper, J.P. Ocular lymphoid neoplasms. Am. J. Ophthalmol. 87:614–618, 1979.
12. Cummings, N.A., Schall, G.L., Asofsky, R., Anderson, L.G., Talal, N. Sjögren's syndrome-newer aspects of research, diagnosis and therapy. Ann. Intern. Med. 75:937, 1971.
13. Feltkamp, T.E.W., van Rossun, A.L. Antibodies to salivary duct cells, and other autoantibodies in patients with Sjögren's syndrome and other idiopathic autoimmune diseases. Clin. Exp. Immunol. 3:1, 1968.
14. Chused, T.M., Kassan, S.S., Opelz, G., Moutsopoulos, H.M., Terasaki, P.I. Sjögren's syndrome associated with HLA-Dw3. N. Engl. J. Med. 296:895, 1977.
15. Friedlander, M.H. Allergy and Immunology of the Eye. Harper and Row, Hagerstown, 1979, p. 231.
16. Leventhal, B.G., Waldorf, D.S., Tallal, N. Impaired lymphocyte transformation and delayed hypersensitivity in Sjögren's syndrome. J. Clin. Invest. 46:133, 1967.
17. Kessler, H.S. A laboratory model for Sjögren's syndrome. Am. J. Pathol. 52:671, 1968.

18. Kessler, H.S., Cubberly, M., Manski, W. Eye changes in the autoimmune NZB and NZB × NZW mice. Arch. Ophthalmol. 85:211, 1971.

19. Tabbarra, K.F. Alternate-day steroid therapy in patients with Sjögren's syndrome. Invest. Ophthalmol. Vis. Sci. 18 (Suppl.):70, April 1979.

20. Scharf, J.M., Obedeance, N., Meskulam, T., Nahir, M., Merzbach, D., Scharf, J.A., Zones, S. Influence of bromhexine on tear lysozyme level in keratoconjunctivitis. Am. J. Ophthalmol. 92:21–23, 1981.

CHAPTER ELEVEN

Tumor Immunology

IMMUNOLOGICAL SURVEILLANCE

In 1908, Paul Ehrlich,[1] the famous biologist, postulated that cancer cells arise frequently and that they can be recognized as foreign antigens by the host. Fifty years later, Lewis Thomas[2] suggested that the immunological system itself may have developed in order to police the body for altered cells which become neoplastic. This policing action is called immunological surveillance.

While a number of investigators have demonstrated that the immune surveillance hypothesis cannot adequately explain all aspects of the host tumor mechanism, it is nevertheless a useful theoretical construct to aid the nonimmunologist in understanding tumor immunology.

An imbalance in the surveillance mechanism of the host immune system is therefore thought to be involved in the development of tumors. A tumor cell represents a foreign configuration to the host in which it arises. The immune mechanisms operable against tumor cells are the same as those marshalled in response to any other foreign configuration.

This concept of immunological surveillance is supported by the clinically observed higher incidence of malignancy in patients with immunological deficiency syndromes or immune suppression secondary to drugs.[3]

For reasons thus far unclear, some cells escape this mechanism with subsequent development of tumors. Tumor growth in the face of supposedly protective immune mechanisms is called immunological escape.

In order for the immunological surveillance mechanism to operate, cancer cells must display new surface antigens which can be recognized by the host immune cells. The following section describes tumor antigens.

TUMOR ANTIGENS

Antigens arise in tumors as a consequence of neoplastic changes and are specific for each tumor or group of tumors. These antigens are referred to as tumor-specific transplantation antigens (TSTA) or tumor-specific antigens (TSA). These cell membrane antigens are mainly responsible for a cell-mediated immune response analogous to a homograft reaction (which is why it is called a tumor-specific transplantation antigen). The origins of the newly acquired antigens are influenced by the oncogenic or cancer-inducing agent.[4] A classification of tumor antigens follows.

1. Virus-induced antigens (virus-coded). These include oncogenic DNA viruses and oncogenic RNA viruses. Where the malignancy is of viral origin, the cell membrane antigens reflect the causative virus, regardless of the animal species or tissue harboring the neoplasm. There is then cross-reactivity.[5]

2. Chemical carcinogen-induced tumor antigens (host coded). These chemical agents induce unique tumor-specific antigens which seem to develop by alteration of the host genes. Therefore, resistance to one chemically induced tumor does not prevent growth of a second tumor. Since these antigens are always unique for a given tumor and show no cross-reactivity, the production of a specific immune therapy becomes more difficult. For example, if a single mouse is painted with methylcholanthrene in several different areas, each of the resulting

carcinomas will express cell-surface antigens that are identical on all cells within that tumor but different from the antigens expressed by the other chemically induced tumors.[6]

3. Illegitimate antigens. There is evidence of reversion, or failure to suppress genes from an embryonic state, in some forms of malignancy. These antigens are called oncofetal. These fetal antigens are found on the surface of tumor cells but are easily shed into the environment. The most widely studied fetal antigens are carcinoembryonic antigen (CEA) and alpha-fetoprotein. CEA is useful in the diagnosis and monitoring of patients with tumors of the gastrointestinal tract. Alpha-fetoprotein is detectable in patients with hepatomas and embryonal carcinoma. Another type of illegitimate antigen occurs when normal tissue antigen appears on the wrong tissue.[7]

HOST IMMUNE RESPONSES

Tumor antigens can provoke a variety of immune responses in experimental animals. Both cellular and humoral immunity can be detected, directed specifically at cell surface antigens of tumor cells.

Circulating antibody can be clearly cytotoxic for tumors which persist in the form of isolated cells, but other cellular mechanisms would seem to be needed for the onslaught against a solid tumor. Indeed, three kinds of killer cells seem to be involved in cell-mediated immunity to tumors[8]: T-cells, natural killer cells (NK), and K, or killer cells, which are responsible for antibody dependent, cell-mediated cytotoxicity (ADCC) (Fig. 11.1).

As mentioned above, tumor growth in the face of these immune mechanisms is termed immunological escape. The various mechanisms of immunological es-

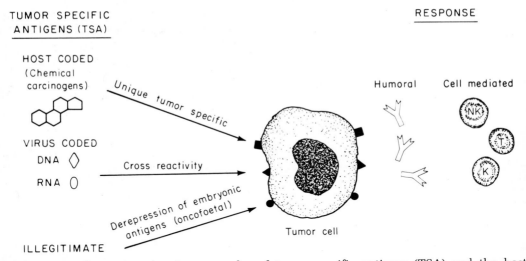

Figure 11.1 Illustration showing examples of tumor-specific antigens (TSA) and the host response to them. 1) Chemical carcinogens result in antigens which are coded by the genetic material of the host. They result in tumors with unique tumor specific cell-surface antigens which show no cross-reactivity. 2) Virus-induced tumors have tumor specific antigens coded by the virus so that each tumor induced by a single virus will have the same TSA on the cell surface and show cross-reactivity. 3) Illegitimate antigens represent antigens which appear at the wrong time from what is thought to represent a failure to suppress (a derepression) embryonic antigens. They are called oncofetal antigens. The immune response to these antigens involves both humoral and cell-mediated components. The cell-mediated immune (CMI) response is considered more important. There are at least three kinds of killer cells involved in the cell-mediated response to tumors—the T-cell, the natural killer (NK) cell, and the K or killer cell responsible for the ADCC mechanism. The question of which effector cell is more important remains unknown. Tumor growth in the face of these immune mechanisms is termed immunological escape.

cape are beyond the scope of this book. Suffice it to say that overt cancer develops if for any reason the immunological surveillance mechanism is defective. Again, this is supported by the observation that malignant disease is more prevalent in patients who have undergone organ transplantation and are immunosuppressed or in patients who have congenital immune deficiency diseases. In addition, it is a common experience that cell-mediated immunity, as shown by cutaneous reactivity to a variety of antigens, is usually depressed in a nonspecific manner in patients with malignant disease.

There are three general areas of investigation involving the immunology of tumors: 1) the study of immune responses by an organism to a tumor; 2) the development of immunodiagnostic assays as a method to detect the early presence of tumor formation; and 3) the development of specific immunotherapeutic agents directed against tumors. All of these areas of investigation are still in early stages. The following section on ocular tumors describes some of the findings.

OCULAR TUMORS

Malignant melanoma of the uveal tract is the most common primary intraocular tumor.

Antitumor antibodies or tumor-associated antibodies (TAA) have been shown to be present in the sera of patients harboring a small primary melanoma. They are not found with larger tumors. Their role is unclear. They are thought to appear as a result of destruction of tumor cells rather than as a protection of the host from metastases. Cellular reactivity to TAA can be demonstrated in patients with uveal melanomas by use of the leukocyte migration inhibition assay. This in vitro assay has been used to distinguish choroidal melanomas from similarly appearing choroidal lesions.[10]

Another immunodiagnostic assay is the presence or absence of the oncofetal antigen, carcinoembryonic antigen (CEA), found in association with endodermally derived malignancies such as colon tumors. The finding of a positive CEA suggests that a choroidal mass is not due to a

melanoma.[11] At present, immunotherapy for choroidal melanoma is an experimental procedure of undetermined therapeutic efficacy.

Zimmerman and associates[12] have concluded, on an epidemiological basis, that removal of an eye with a choroidal melanoma results in a greater incidence of mortality due to an immune protective effect of the presence of the tumor. It is postulated that the tumor probably continues to stimulate an immune response and to give some protection against spreading tumor formation. This concept is controversial.

Retinoblastoma is the most common intraocular malignancy of childhood. The high rate of spontaneous regression of this tumor has led to speculation that immunological factors are particularly important in this tumor.

As in other kinds of tumors, the cell-mediated immune response to tumor-associated antigens is thought to be important in resistance to retinoblastomas. Higher levels of cytotoxicity against tissue culture lines from retinoblastoma patients can be found when compared to controls.[13] The meaning of this finding remains unclear, as does the exact antigen resulting in the response.

If retinoblastoma tumor cells are injected into the anterior chamber of athymic "nude" mice, which possess a severe defect in cellular immunity, the tumor grows in some of these animals.[14]

An increasingly important immunodiagnostic assay is the serum level of immune complexes. In some tumors, such as the retinoblastoma, immune complexes [consisting of (TAA) and antibodies] are elevated. These immune complexes are thought to block the host's cell-mediated immunological response toward tumor antigens and the serum levels may be of importance in correlating disease status, presence of metastases, and prognosis.[15]

REFERENCES

1. Weissman, I.L., Hood, L., Wood, W.B. Essential Concepts in Immunology. The Benjamin/Cummings Publishing Co., Inc., Menlo Park, California, 1978, p. 137.
2. Thomas, L., Lawrence, H.S. Cellular and Hu-

moral Aspects of the Hypersensitive State. Hoeber, New York, 1959, p. 529.

3. Waldmann, T.A., Strober, W., Blaese, R.M. Immunodeficiency disease and malignancy. Various immunologic deficiencies of man and the role of immune processes in the control of malignant disease. Ann. Intern. Med. 77:605–628, 1972.

4. Smith, R.I. Tumor specific immune mechanisms. N. Engl. J. Med. 287:439, 1972.

5. Winters, W.D. Immunovirology. In Cancer, Epidemiology and Prevention edited by Shottenfield, D. Charles C Thomas, Springfield, 1975, pp. 207–230.

6. Wilson, R.E., Alexander, P., Rosenberg, S.A., Simmons, R.L. Horizons in tumor immunology. A seminar. Arch. Surg. 109:17–29, 1974.

7. Khoo, S.K., Warner, N.I., Lie, J.T., MacKay, I.R. Carcinoembryonic antigenic activity of tissue extracts. A quantitative study of malignant and benign neoplasms, cirrhotic liver, normal adult and fetal organs. Int. J. Cancer 11:681–687, 1973.

8. Perlmann, P., O'Tolle, G., Unsgaard, B. Cell-mediated immune mechanisms of tumor cell destruction. Fed. Proc. 32:153–155, 1973.

9. Wong, I.G., Oskvig, R.M. Immunofluorescent detection of antibodies to ocular melanomas. Arch. Ophthalmol. 92:98, 1974.

10. Char, D.H. Inhibition of leukocyte migration with melanoma-associated antigens in choroidal tumors. Invest. Ophthalmol. Vis. Sci. 16:176, 1977.

11. Tormey, D.C., Waalkes, T.P., Snyder, J.J., Simon, R.M. Biological markers in breast carcinoma III. Clinical correlations with carcinoembryonic antigen. Cancer 39:2397, 1977.

12. Zimmerman, L.E., Mclean, I.W., Foster, W.D. Does enucleation of the eye containing a malignant melanoma prevent or accelerate the dissemination of tumour cells? Br. J. Ophthalmol. 62:420–425, 1978.

13. Char, D.H., Ellsworth, R., Rabson, A.S., Albert, D.M., Herbeman, R.B. Cell-mediated immunity to a retinoblastoma tissue culture line in patients with retinoblastoma. Am. J. Ophthalmol. 78:5, 1974.

14. Gallie, B.L., Albert, D.M., Wong, J.J.Y., Buyukmichi, N., Puliafito, C.A. Heterotransplantation of retinoblastoma into the athymice "nude" mouse. Invest. Ophthalmol. 16:256, 1977.

15. Char, D.H., Christensen, M., Goldberg, L., Stein, P. Immune complexes in retinoblastoma. Am. J. Ophthalmol. 86:395–399, 1978.

CHAPTER TWELVE

Glossary

ADAPTIVE (SPECIFIC) IMMUNITY: A phylogenetically more recently evolved system which results in the production of specific antibodies to the immunogen and a cell-mediated immune response. When compared to the nonspecific primary response, adaptive immunity requires longer to develop, has highly specific effector systems, and expresses memory.

ADCC (antibody-dependent cellular cytotoxicity): Target cells coated with IgG antibody may be destroyed by certain cells, such as K-cells or macrophages.

ADJUVANT: Certain substances capable of enhancing the immune response when injected with an antigen.

AGGLUTININ: An antibody which produces aggregation, or agglutination of a particle or an insoluble antigen.

ALLERGEN: A specific type of antigen or immunogen, capable of inducing an allergic (hypersensitivity) reaction.

ALLERGY: An acquired hypersensitivity, which results in damage to host tissues. This is a reaction mediated by IgE antibodies. Implied in the definition is the fact that the foreign substance is usually innocuous, and its source is from the external environment, e.g., pollens.

ALLOGRAFT (HOMOGRAFT): Histoincompatible (has different histocompatibility antigens than self) but of the same species. For example, a corneal graft from one individual transplanted to another is an allogeneic graft or an allograft. An immune reaction to this graft would be an allograft reaction.

ALTERNATE PATHWAY: A mechanism of complement activation through bacterial products such as endotoxin or aggregated IgA and that does not require antibody.

ANAMNESTIC RESPONSE: Re-exposure to an antigen previously encountered that results in an accelerated production of antibody.

ANAPHYLATOXIN: Small cleavage products of the complement cascade which have anaphylatoxic activities. Specifically, the peptides C3a and C5a can cause contraction of smooth muscle, increased vascular permeability, and release of histamine from mast cells.

ANAPHYLAXIS: An immediate hypersensitivity response involving IgE and occurring within minutes of re-exposure to an antigen, resulting in the release of pharmacologically active substances from mast cells.

ANTIBODIES (Ab): Immunoglobulin proteins produced by B-lymphocytes in response to antigenic stimulation. Antibody combines specifically with the inducing antigen. There are five classes of antibodies or immunoglobulins.

ANTIGEN (Ag): A foreign substance with the capacity to evoke an immunological response. The antigenic determinant is that three-dimensional part of an antigen molecule with which an antibody can combine.

ANTILYMPHOCYTE SERUM (ALS): An antiserum against lymphocytes produced by the injection of an animal with lymphocytes. This antiserum kills lymphocytes and is thus immunosuppressive.

ANTINUCLEAR FACTORS: In systemic lupus erythematosus (SLE), the leukocyte nucleus may undergo denaturation and phagocytosis because of an antibody directed against a component of the nucleus. The first antinuclear factor discovered was directed against deoxyribonucleoprotein and is responsible for the lupus erythematosus (LE) cell phenomenon. Antinuclear factors have also been found against other components of the leukocyte nucleus.

ARTHUS REACTION: The injection of antigen into an animal possessing circulating antibodies to that antigen results, clinically, in an edematous, hemorrhagic, and necrotic lesion at the site of injection. Histologically, an acute inflammatory reaction with vascular occlusion and an accumulation of neutrophils is observed. A type III hypersensitivity reaction.

ATOPY: Genetically predisposed to type I allergic reactions.

AUER REACTION: The tendency of vessels injured by nonimmune damage in one part of the body to become more permeable with subsequent immune (Ag-Ab) reactions in other parts of the body. This has been postulated as occurring in recurrent iritis.

AUTOANTIBODY: The production of antibodies which react against one's own antigens.

AUTOGRAFT: Graft tissue derived from the same individual to whom it is being transplanted.

AUTOIMMUNE DISEASE: A response of autoantibodies, or immune competent cells, directed against the patient's own antigens, with resulting damage to tissues. Autoimmunity may also be considered a tertiary manifestation of the immune response directed against antigens whose inappropriate processing leads to destruction of normal tissue. The latter differs from the classical concept of a primary attack of the host against its own tissue.

AUTOIMMUNE RESPONSE: An autoantibody response directed to a "self-antigen," or reactivity of lymphocytes sensitized to a "self-antigen." The autoimmune response may or may not be associated with autoimmune disease.

AUTOLOGOUS: Of self.

BASOPHIL: A granulocyte classified as a mediator cell in immune reactions. After fixation of the cell with homocytotropic antibody (IgE) in combination with an appropriate antigen, the basophil releases chemical substances (mediators) active in type I (anaphylactic) reactions.

BLOCKING ANTIBODY: An antibody which competes locally, or in the circulation, for an antigen and prevents the reaction with homocytotropic antibody fixed to mediator cells. In serum, these are mainly IgG antibodies and may be induced by repeated injections of antigen.

B-LYMPHOCYTE (B-CELL): Effector cell for the humoral immune response. "B" refers to the site of presumed differentiation of these cells: the Bursa of Fabricius, the cloacal structure in birds which contains the cellular elements responsible for differentiation of these cells. The bursal equivalent in humans may be gut-associated lymphoid tissue, fetal liver, or bone marrow.

BURSA OF FABRICIUS: See B-lymphocyte.

CELL-MEDIATED IMMUNITY: That arm of the adaptive immune response which is mediated by T-lymphocytes (T-cells) and can only be transferred by these cells. A delayed hypersensitivity reaction (tuberculin response) is an example.

CLASSICAL PATHWAY: The mechanism of complement activation which involves antigen-antibody interaction.

Only IgG and IgM have F_c receptors which will bind complement and initiate the complement cascade.

CLONE: A population of cells derived from a single cell.

CLONAL SELECTION THEORY: Proposes that an immunologically responsive cell contains genetic information to respond to a single antigen even before the cell encounters it. The lymphocyte population of an individual is preprogrammed to contain a diverse library of cells which respond to various antigens. The encounter between the antigen and the precommitted cell results in clonal expansion: the proliferation and generation of many similar cells producing the same antibody.

COMPLEMENT (C): Originally implied an auxiliary factor in the serum that acted on an antibody-coated cell to result in lysis of that cell. Complement is now known to be a sequence or cascade of at least 21 serum proteins that react in a sequential fashion to amplify an immune reaction and can result in cell membrane damage if it proceeds to the final steps. Other functions of activated complement include chemotaxis, immune adherence and anaphylatoxin activity.

CYCLIC NUCLEOTIDE SYSTEM (SECOND MESSENGER SYSTEM): A system of cell membrane enzymes which acts as receptors for primary messengers, or hormones, of the autonomic nervous system. Stimulation of guanylate cyclase by the parasympathetic system results in production of cyclic guanosine monophosphate (cGMP). Stimulation of adenyl cyclase by the sympathetic system results in production of cyclic adenosine monophosphate (cAMP). cGMP and cAMP act as second messengers and control certain cell functions.

CYTOTROPIC ANTIBODIES: Antibodies that have the property of binding or fixing to certain cells. For example, IgE has a strong tendency to bind to mast cells, or basophils. The binding is through the F_c region of the antibody to an F_c receptor on the cell.

DELAYED HYPERSENSITIVITY: On re-exposure to antigen, this reaction requires 24 to 48 hours to develop. It is mediated by T-cells and not antibody and can only be transferred by T-cells. The response to tuberculin is an example.

DESENSITIZATION: The process of reducing immediate hypersensitivity to an allergen by treating with minute but increasing amounts of the antigen over a prolonged period of time. This is thought to work by inducing blocking antibodies.

ENDOTOXIN: An integral part of the cell wall of gram-negative organisms. It is composed of a lipid polysaccharide complex. The toxicity resides in the phospholipid fraction, the immunogenicity in the polysaccharide fraction. Endotoxins are detected in the Shwartzman reaction.

ENHANCEMENT: The condition where antibody protects an antigen from destruction by a cytotoxic cell. The antibody conceals the antigen from recognition and destruction by cytotoxic cells.

EOSINOPHIL: A granulocyte recruited to the site of inflammation by products released by mast cells and basophils. Eosinophils contain chemicals that can neutralize or modulate the effects of products released by the mediator cells during hypersensitivity reactions.

EOSINOPHILIC CHEMOTACTIC FACTOR OF ANAPHYLAXIS (ECF-A): The tetrapeptide released by mast cells and basophils which attracts eosinophils.

EXOTOXIN: Soluble molecules elaborated by bacteria as extracellular products that have the capacity to act as cell poisons. They bind to tissue and induce antibodies (antitoxin). The exotoxins can be altered (denatured) to form toxoids, substances that retain their immunogenicity but lose their toxicity.

F$_{ab}$ (FRAGMENT ANTIGEN BINDING): The papain fragment of IgG which binds specifically with antigen.

F$_c$ (FRAGMENT CRYSTALLIZABLE): The papain fragment of immunoglobulin IgG which does not bind with antigen. It was found to be crystallizable, and is responsible for many of the other biological properties of antibody, e.g., complement binding, transplacental passage, and attachment to cells.

GRAFT-VERSUS-HOST REACTION (GvH): When competent immune cells are transferred from a donor to a histoincompatible (nontwin) recipient incapable of rejecting them, the grafted cells react immunologically against the host. T-cells mediate the reactivity.

HAPTEN: An antigen, capable of binding with antibody but incapable of inducing an antibody response. Must be bound to a carrier protein to be immunogenic.

HETEROGRAFT (XENOGRAFT): A graft from one species transplanted to another.

HISTAMINE: One of the pharmacologically active mediators of immediate hypersensitivity found in the granules of mast cells, basophils, and platelets. It is responsible for the itching symptom in allergic reactions and causes increased vascular permeability and dilatation.

HISTOCOMPATIBILITY ANTIGENS (TRANSPLANTATION ANTIGENS): The surface glycoproteins on cells which give an organ its recognizable antigenicity and evokes the rejection phenomenon.

HOMOCYTOTROPIC ANTIBODY: See Cytotropic Antibody

HLA (HUMAN LEUKOCYTE ANTIGENS): Cell surface antigens coded for by a small, complex genetic region on chromosome 6 in humans. This is the major histocompatibility complex in humans and has special importance be-

cause of the relationship of certain HLA antigens to human diseases. This genetic region also probably determines cellular interactions in an immune response to foreign antigens.

IMMUNE ADHERENCE: The increased adherence of antigen/antibody to phagocytes through a complement receptor in these cells. Responsible for increased phagocytosis.

IMMUNE COMPLEX DISEASE: Freely circulating antigen that combines with specific antibodies can form immune complexes. These complexes lodge on blood vessel basement membranes where they activate complement and initiate a response consisting of phagocytosis and inflammation. This usually results in their elimination. However, if antigen persists or complexes are not removed, chronic or recurrent inflammatory disease may result.

IMMUNE RESPONSE: The production of a nonspecific response or specific antibodies and cell-mediated immunity subsequent to introduction of a foreign substance into a host.

IMMUNOGEN: See Antigen.

IMMUNOGLOBULIN: See Antibodies.

IMMUNOLOGICAL ESCAPE: The ability of tumors to escape immune response by host-determined immune mechanisms.

IMMUNOLOGICAL PRIVILEGE: The persistence of foreign antigen in a host based on unique anatomic, physiological, or biochemical features.

IMMUNOLOGICAL SURVEILLANCE: Theoretically, cancer cells arise frequently during the lifetime of the host. Immunological surveillance is thought to be responsible for recognizing these cells as foreign (because of new antigens expressed on these cells) and rejecting them.

IMMUNOLOGICAL TOLERANCE: Specific unresponsiveness to a foreign substance. It may be due to suppressor cells or to the elimination of the responding clone of lymphocytes.

IMMUNOLOGICALLY MEDIATED DISEASE (IMD): Persistance of antigen can lead to tissue damage in the host caused by normal immunological reactions.

IMMUNOMODULATION: The stimulation or suppression of the immune responsiveness of a host.

IMMUNOPOTENTIATOR: A substance which increases or augments certain aspects of the immune response.

IMMUNOSUPPRESSION: The inhibition, usually nonspecifically, of immune responsiveness.

INTERFERON: A protein produced by a wide variety of cells following viral infection or after exposure to certain inducers. Also, a lymphokine produced by lymphoid cells on exposure to certain antigens or re-exposure to these antigens. Interferon induces an antiviral protein in uninfected cells. Interferon also augments NK.

ISOGRAFT (ISOGENEIC or SYNGENEIC): Histocompatible, as with identical twins. Also found with highly inbred strains of mice. There is close to 100% survival of transplanted grafts since there is almost 100% genetic compatibility.

KILLER LYMPHOCYTES (K-CELLS): See ADCC.

KININS: Small peptides with strong vasoactive properties that result from a sequential enzymatic breakdown of a plasma protein precursor, Kallikrein. The kinin system is one of the biological amplification systems in plasma which augment the inflammatory reaction.

LYMPHOCYTE: Lymphoid cells of the immune system can react specifically with antigen, and elaborate cell products. There are two types, which are classified on the basis of their site of differentiation into thymus-derived (T-cell) and bursa-derived (B-cell). Since their appearance is similar by light microscopy, they must be differentiated by surface markers. B-cells can be identified by the presence of antibody on the cell surface, and T-cells can be identified by the presence of human T-lymphocyte antigen on their cell surface. All other lymphoid cells are referred to as null cells.

LYMPHOKINES: The products of lymphocytes (T-cells) which modulate other T-cell and macrophage functions. These chemical messengers are required for the cell-mediated immune response.

MACROPHAGE: Large phagocytic cells required for humoral and cell-mediated immune response (processes and presents antigen). Also, an effector cell of the cell-mediated immune response.

MAST CELL: A tissue-bound mediator cell with functions similar to those of blood-borne basophil. After fixation of the cell with homocytotropic antibody (IgE), in combination with an appropriate antigen, the mast cell releases chemical substances active in type I (anaphylactic) reactions.

MEDIATOR CELL: Cells which release chemical substances (mediators) with a variety of biological activities, such as causing changes in vascular permeability and chemotaxis. Mediator cells include mast cells, basophils, platelets, enterochromatin cells, and neutrophils.

MEMORY CELLS: Helper T-cells, which, on second exposure to antigen, proliferate and induce a rapid and strong immunological response.

MONOCLONAL ANTIBODY FORMATION: The production of monospecific antibody by hybridizing a single antibody-producing cell to a myeloma (cancer) cell. The hybrid produces large quantities of the specific antibody.

NATURAL KILLER CELL (NK): Recognizes tumor and virus infected cells as nonself and causes their lysis. Requires no previous experience with antigen.

ONCOFETAL ANTIGENS: Antigens normally expressed during fetal development but not by differentiated cells. These antigens are often expressed on tumor cells.

OPSONIZATION: The increased adherence of particulate antigens to phagocytic cells caused by specific antibody. This results in enhanced phagocytosis.

OPSONINS: Antibodies which cause opsonization.

PLASMA CELLS: A lymphoid cell that matures from the B-lymphocyte series into an antibody-producing cell.

PLATELET ACTIVATING FACTOR (PAF): A low molecular weight mediator released by mast cells and basophils, inducing platelet aggregation and secretion.

PRAUSNITZ-KÜSTNER (P-K) TEST: Atopic sensitivity can be assessed by the response to an intradermal challenge with antigen. The release of histamine and other mediators rapidly produces a wheal and erythema. The responsible IgE antibody can be demonstrated by the ability of the allergic patient's serum to passively sensitize the skin of normal subjects. Serum from a sensitized individual is injected intradermally into a normal recipient. After a period of several days, antigen is injected in the same site, and the response is evaluated.

PROSTAGLANDINS: Prostaglandins are a family of biologically active lipids present in most tissues and released upon damage to that tissue. In the eye, they cause a dramatic increase in the protein of the aqueous humor.

RHEUMATOID FACTOR (Rhf): Antibodies of various classes directed against antigenic sites on the F_c portion of the heavy chain of immunoglobulin G. Rheumatoid factor is thus an autoantibody. Rheumatoid factor forms the basis of the sheep agglutination test and the latex fixation test for rheumatoid arthritis.

SECRETORY COMPONENT (SC): A unique structure synthesized in epithelial cells and added to an IgA molecule as it is transported across a mucous membrane. SC appears to protect the antibody against enzymatic degradation and fixes it to the mucosa.

SHWARTZMAN REACTION: The reaction produced by the subcutaneous injection of bacterial endotoxin 24 hours after a primary dose. The second injection results in a localized vasculitis and a hemorrhagic necrosis (localized Shwartzman reaction). If the injection is given intravenously, the animal may die in 24 hours (general Shwartzman reaction). Clinically, this is seen in gram-negative sepsis and results in shock, fever, leukopenia, and intravascular coagulation.

SLOW REACTING SUBSTANCE OF ANAPHYLAXIS (SRS-A): This low molecular weight (500 MW) mediator is released from mast cells and basophils during a type I reaction. In general, the biological activity of SRS-A is similar to histamine, but develops more slowly and lasts longer.

T-LYMPHOCYTE (T-CELL): Thymus-derived lymphocyte that mediates cellular immunity and modulates the immune response through suppressor and helper cells.

TUMOR-SPECIFIC ANTIGENS (TSA): Antigens on tumors which are specific for each tumor or group of tumors. The cell membrane antigens may be responsible for a cell-mediated immune response resulting in its rejection (similar to graft rejection). These antigens are therefore sometimes referred to as tumor specific transplantation antigens

(TSTA). These antigens depend on the oncogenic, or cancer inducing agent.

TUMOR-ASSOCIATED ANTIBODY (TAA): Antibody directed against tumor antigens may be found in sera of patients harboring tumors.

TRANSFER FACTOR: An effector molecule, released by a sensitized lymphocyte, with the capacity to transfer delayed hypersensitivity to a nonreactive individual. It is thought to be immunologically specific.

WESSELY RING: A white, peripheral ring in the cornea occurring a week after experimental injection of antigen into a cornea. It arises as a result of systemically formed antibody diffusing into a cornea containing residual antigen from a previous injection. The Wessely phenomenon or ring consists of antigen-antibody and complement complexes and polymorphonuclear leukocytes. A Wessely type ring has been described in patients with antigenic corneal foreign bodies.

Index